SIMPLE RAW FOOD MEALS

by Natalia Clarke

Contents

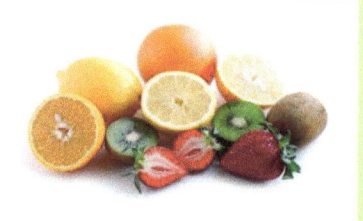

Introduction

I call my food creations **MEALS** rather than **RECIPES** and that is because every creation can serve as a meal depending on the quantity you make. In this book I use no measurements, numbers, times, extensive preparation lists, strange ingredients or special equipment. It is **SIMPLE**. My goal is through introducing simple raw ingredients into your food preparation I would like to encourage you to be creative and adventurous with every meal you have. So what if you don't have kale on a particular day, you might have cucumber, spinach or celery – use that instead. It is not a big disaster. Experiment and be free with your food. Just because something on the list is not in your fridge, doesn't mean you can't make a delicious meal with another ingredient .

3

I provide suggestions for possible replacement foods where appropriate. Tastes differ greatly, as we all know. Some people might like bananas, others are not keen on their texture or smell, therefore, if a meal includes bananas, there is no reason one can't replace it with a pineapple or a mango. It is all about freedom and expressing your creativity through preparing your meals and actively engaging with ingredients. By using your personal taste, creativity and intuition you are sure to come up with some super tasty surprises and vice versa, some meals might not resonate with how you feel on that day. No problem. Next time try something else or make a similar thing, but adjust quantities, sweetness, 'greenness', consistency or replace one fruit for another.

It is in your hands and really simple. That's the beauty and the point of using whole foods in your daily meals. A lot of it is inter changeable.

A lovely friend of mine described it very well what many people I come across struggle with. There is that stumbling block of, on one hand, needing exact lists and instructions and, on the other hand, finding those lists and instructions very restrictive, precise and requiring a fair amount of preparation, which then raises stress levels in many and stops creativity flowing. My friend gave me an example of having cucumber, celery and apple at her disposal, but she didn't know what to do with it. That's exactly the situation I would like you to explore.

The answer is to put the whole lot in your juicer and enjoy. Simple. Do not over think and over complicate the process, but because we are used to a certain way of thinking, behaving and doing things, we often get stuck in that process of making everything harder than it should be. I know exactly what that feels like and, therefore, I am throwing all the rules out of the window with this book of meals. I want my audience to start experimenting and creating the meals, which are just right for them, not because I say you do it a certain way, but because it is something you create yourself, it comes from you and you have a desire to try something new, go on a food adventure and allow yourself to break free.

What's in the book

All my meals are simple to prepare and will be on your plate ready to enjoy in minutes. All meals are raw and vegan. Recipes are inter changeable and can be adapted to your tastes and daily preferences. Enjoy fruit meals, smoothies, salads, sauces, dressings and soups ideas for every day of the week. In my experience some people stick with a few staple meals and use them all the time, others like more variety. The book is perfect for either to give you ideas on what to prepare with ingredients, which can be mixed, matched and swapped for various textures and flavours. Options for replacements or additions are specified where appropriate.

There is no measuring or weighing involved. I believe in personal experimentation with ingredients and creating the dishes you like. No one being is the same, so here is a chance for you to taste a few meals and adjust to your own preferences, if needed, whether you like something thicker or with more liquid, sweeter or more 'earthy' or 'greener' tasting, it is entirely up to you. Flexibility and experimentation are your friends when it comes to making your meals and raw foods are perfect for that.

The book contains ideas on best morning meals, lunches, snacks and evenings meals on a raw food lifestyle. There is also a couple of sweets you might like to try occasionally.

The book's focus is on low-fat and low sodium food. Meals are low on nuts and contain no oils or salt. Through experimentation I found eating low-fat meals with lots of fruit give me the best energy and levels of well-being. The simpler the better! No ready-made, shop-bought artificial condiments or seasonings are used in any of the recipes and the soul focus is on natural whole foods. Enjoy!

Food List

Here is a list of my staple foods, which I use in my meals. That is all that you will need to make any of the dishes included in this book. An important point to mention is that I eat seasonally whenever possible and I strongly encourage it for optimum health and vitality. From spring through to autumn we grow our own food and it is a wonderful practice to get involved with to become a true master of your food choices.

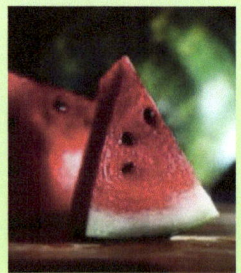

Fruit

- Apples
- Berries (fresh and frozen): strawberries, raspberries, blueberries, blackberries, currents
- Bananas (used in smoothies and post-workout meals especially)
- Dates (used in sauces, sweets and smoothies)
- Red grapes (used in smoothies and in green juices, they combine very well with bitter greens)
- Oranges (mono-meals, smoothies and salad dressings)
- Kiwis
- Mangos
- Papayas
- Pears
- Tangerines/Mandarins
- Lemons
- Avocado
- Tomato

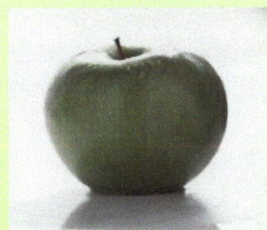

11

Vegetables

- Green/red/yellow peppers
- Green and red cabbage
- Celery
- Courgettes (zucchini)
- Cucumber
- Onions (white/red and spring - optional)
- Beetroot
- Carrot
- Broccoli
- Cauliflower

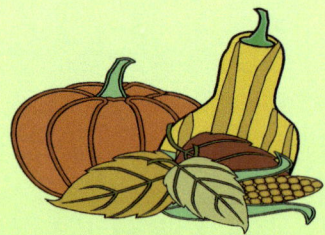

Greens & Herbs

- Lettuces
- Mint
- Parsley
- Dill
- Basil
- Spring Greens
- Kale
- Spinach
- Chard

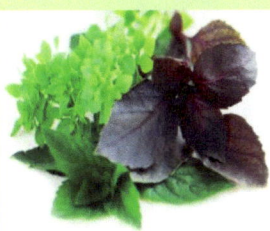

Beans

- Butter beans
- Chickpeas
- Red kidney beans

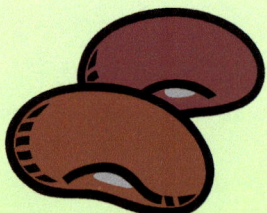

Fats & Super foods

I don't use fats very often and if I do, I keep them to my evening meal. I do sometimes use super foods like chia seeds, carob powder or green powder, but it is absolutely not essential to make or enjoy any of the meals included.

- Flaxseed (for Omega 3)
- Chia seeds (in smoothies and puddings)
- Avocados (for fats)
- Tahini (optional for making hummus)
- Nuts (optional for making sweets, cheeses and snacks) Walnuts, pine nuts
- Carob powder (chocolate replacement)
- Almond butter

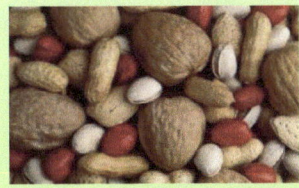

Dried fruit & other

- Raisins
- Apricots
- Oats
- Almond milk
- Coconut water
- Powdered greens (when fresh is not available)

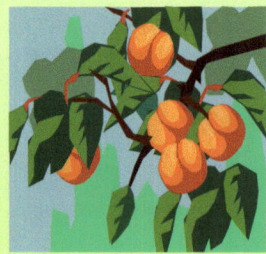

Smoothies & Juices

Enjoy my recipes & pictures of super tasty and nutritious raw drinks

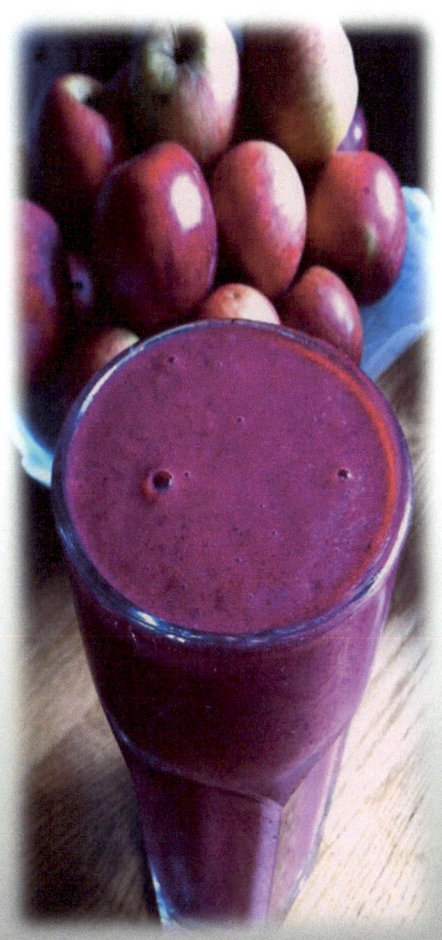

Banana & Date Smoothie

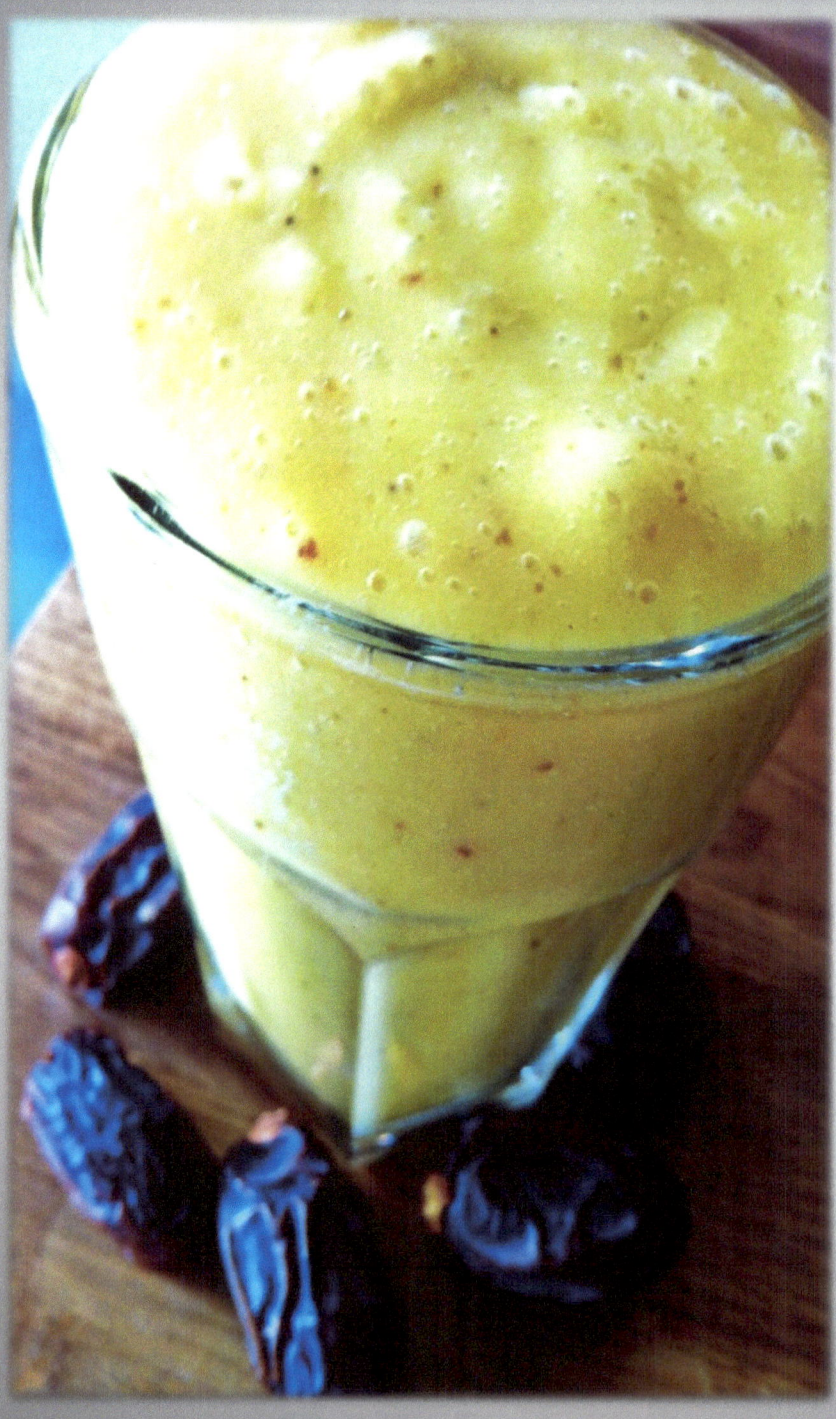

- banana
- dates
- almond milk/water

Mix together in a blender. Can replace banana with either mango or pineapple

Apricot Smoothie

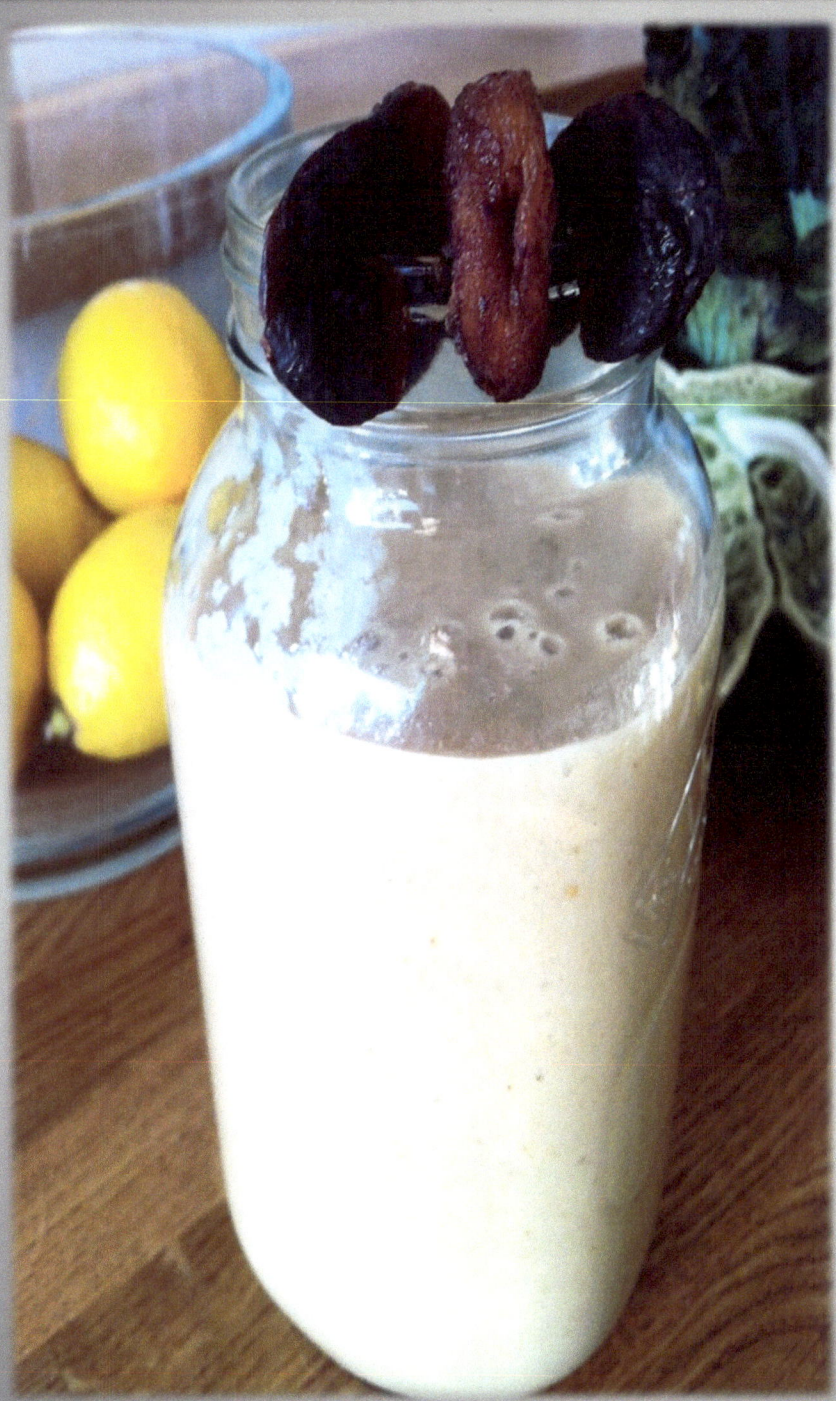

- organic dark dried apricots
- banana
- almond milk

Blend all together. Lovely chilled or with ice

Berries & Dates Smoothie

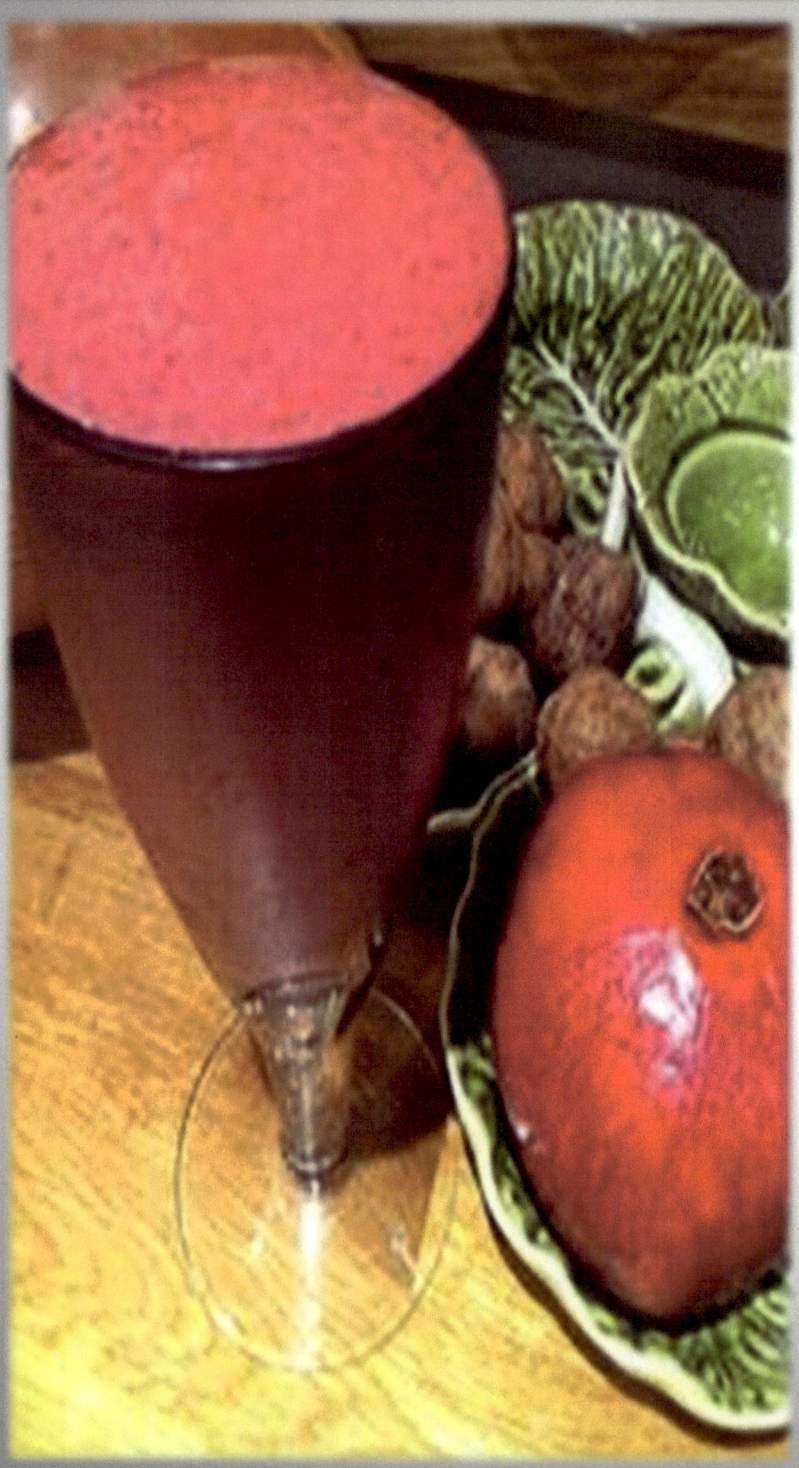

• frozen berries (your choice)
• fresh & frozen banana
• dates
• almond milk or water

In a blender mix all together. Decadent!

Green Thickie

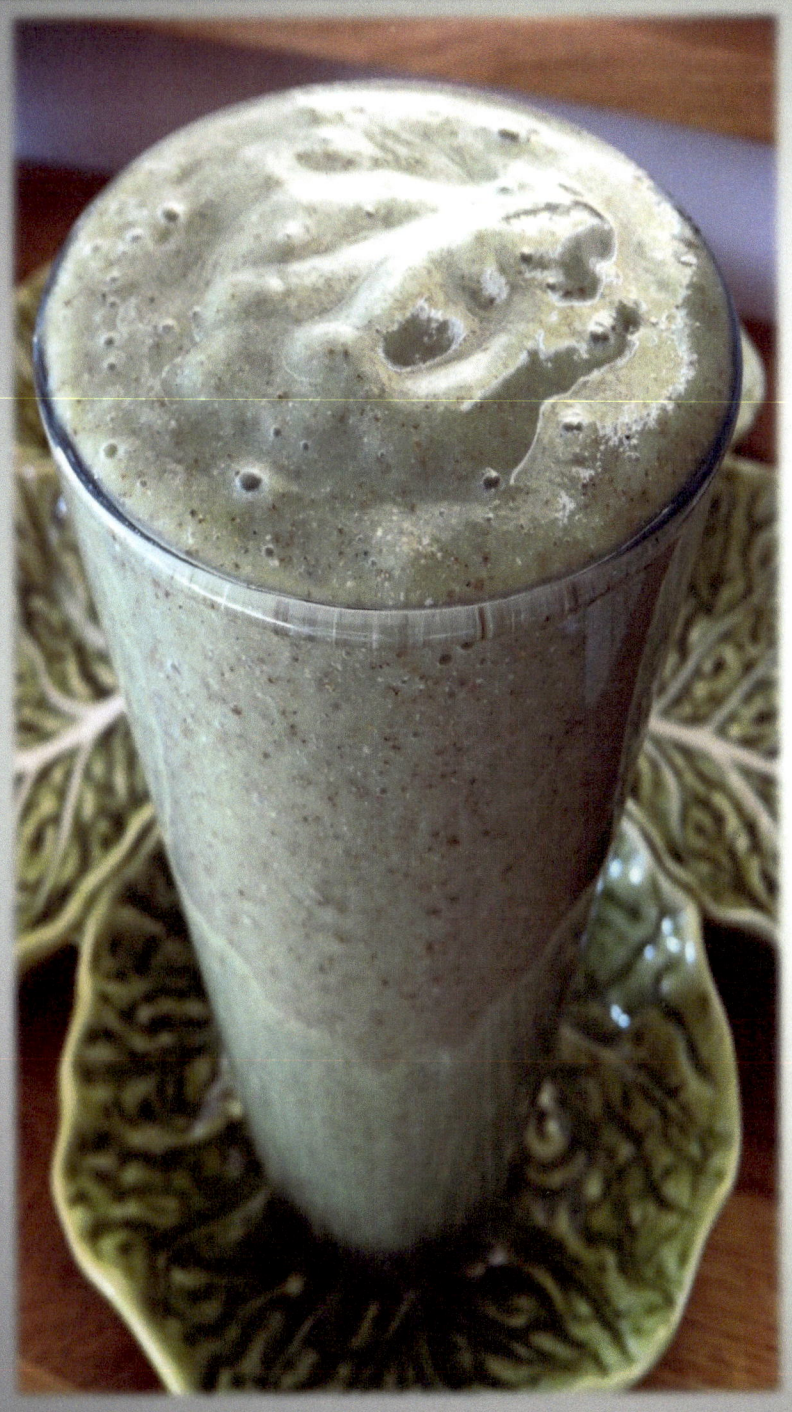

- 2 tbsp chia seeds
- 1 big apple or 2 small ones
- banana (accordng to taste preference)
- 1 tsp powdered greens

Prepare chia seeds by soaking them in water for 30 mins or overnight if you plan to make this smoothie for the morning.

Strawberry Coolie

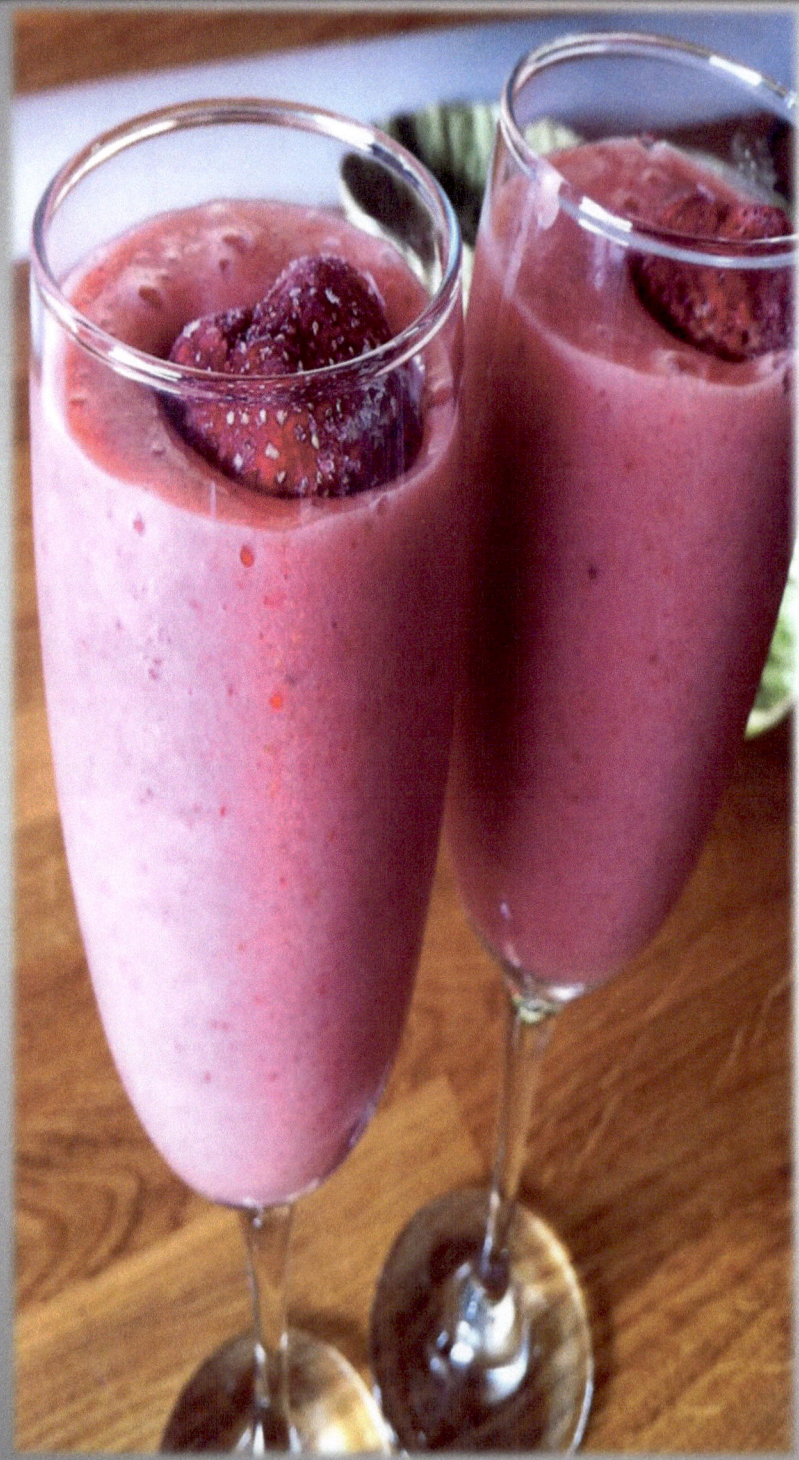

- frozen strawberries
- fresh banana
- frozen banana
- water /nut milk

Blend all together

Blueberry Dream

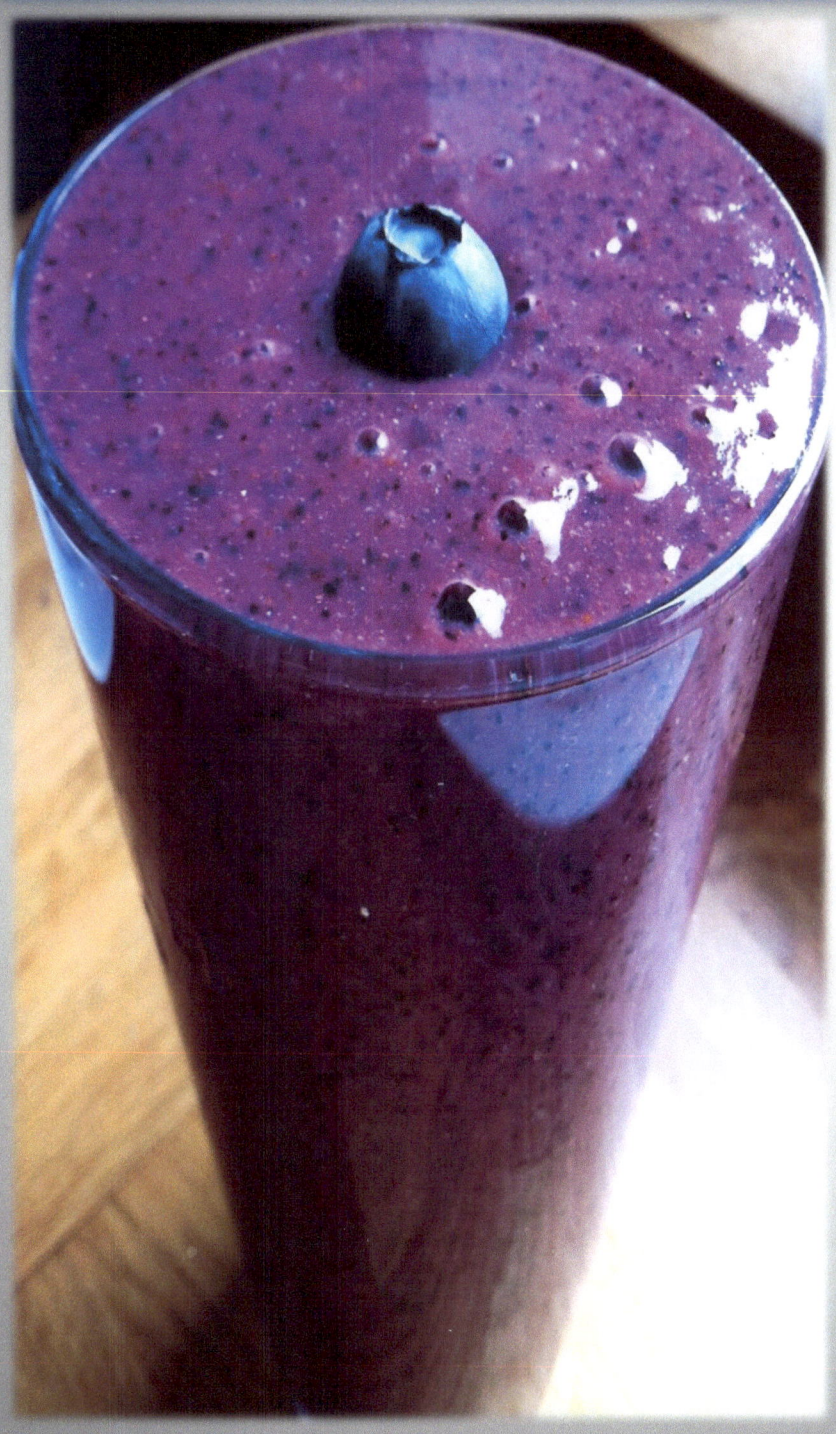

• 350g blueberries or more
• 1 big apple (I like Braeburn variety)
• chia seeds makes it thick (optional)
• water

This Smoothie takes me back to my childhood experience of berry picking in the woods with my parents. Just look at that colour!

Banana & Kale Smoothie

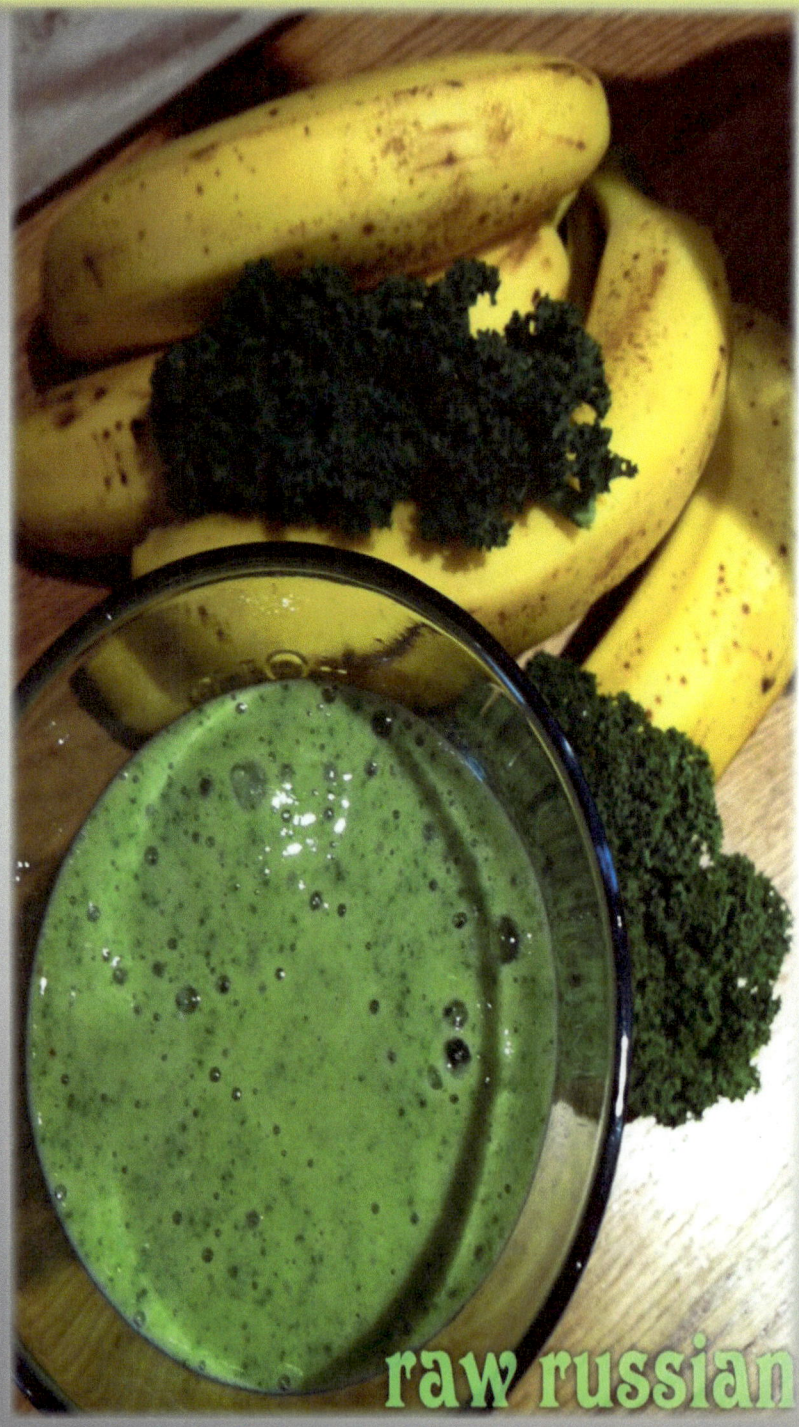

raw russian

- bananas (can replace with mango or pineapple)
- kale
- water or pineapple juice

Use as many or as few bananas as you like depending on how sweet you like your smoothies. The same with kale, use as much or as little as you like depending on how 'green' you like it. Possible substitutes: Replace kale with spinach or even lettuce or celery. You can add parsley/mint to this one too.

Protein Smoothie

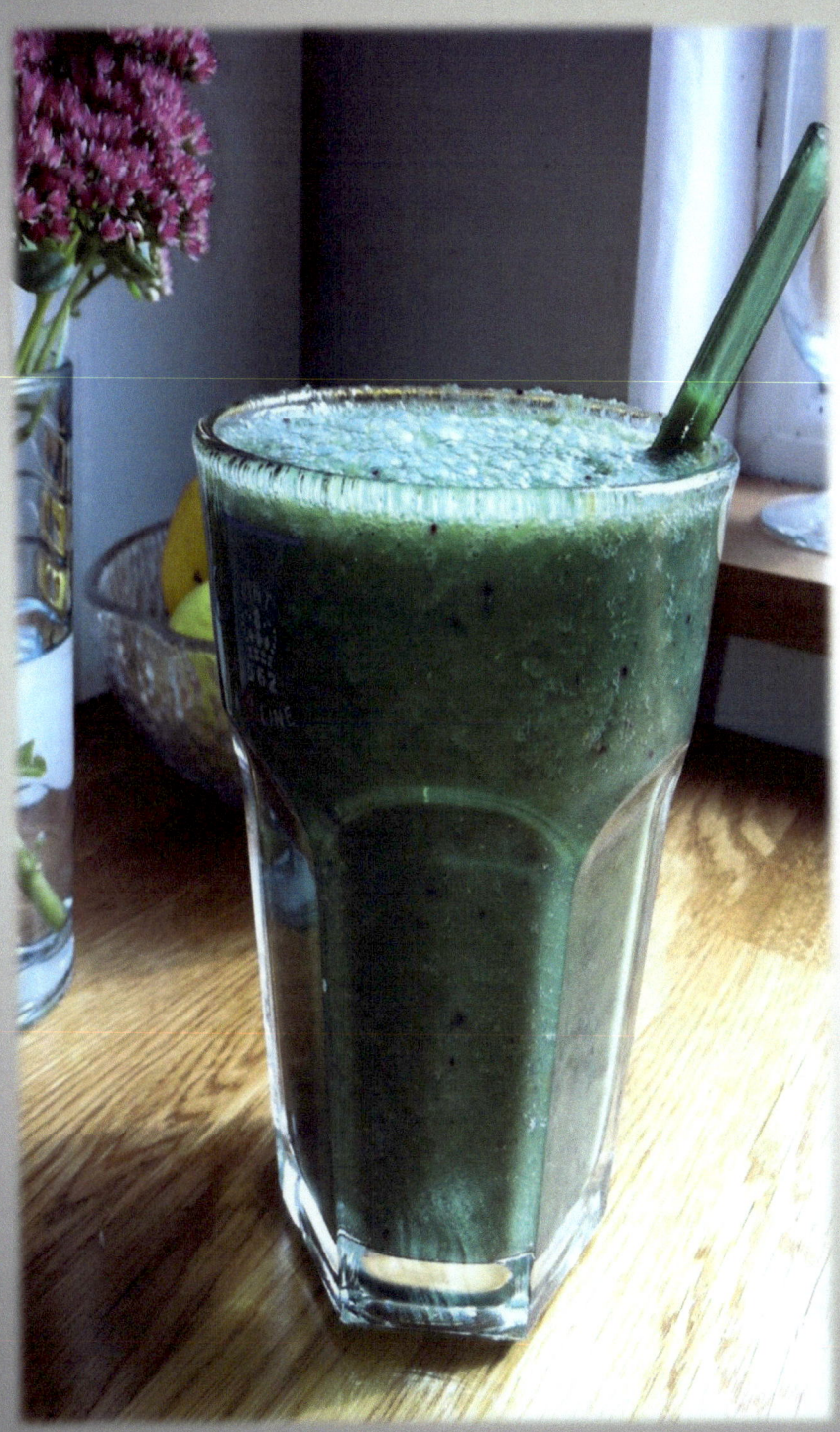

- 1 tbsp Sun Warrior Protein (vanilla flavour)
- spinach (can replace with powdered greens)
- Banana
- 1 orange or satsuma (goes very nicely with vanilla flavour of protein powder)
- coconut water (or just water)
- ice (optional)

Blend all together. Great post-workout meal.

Grape Smoothie

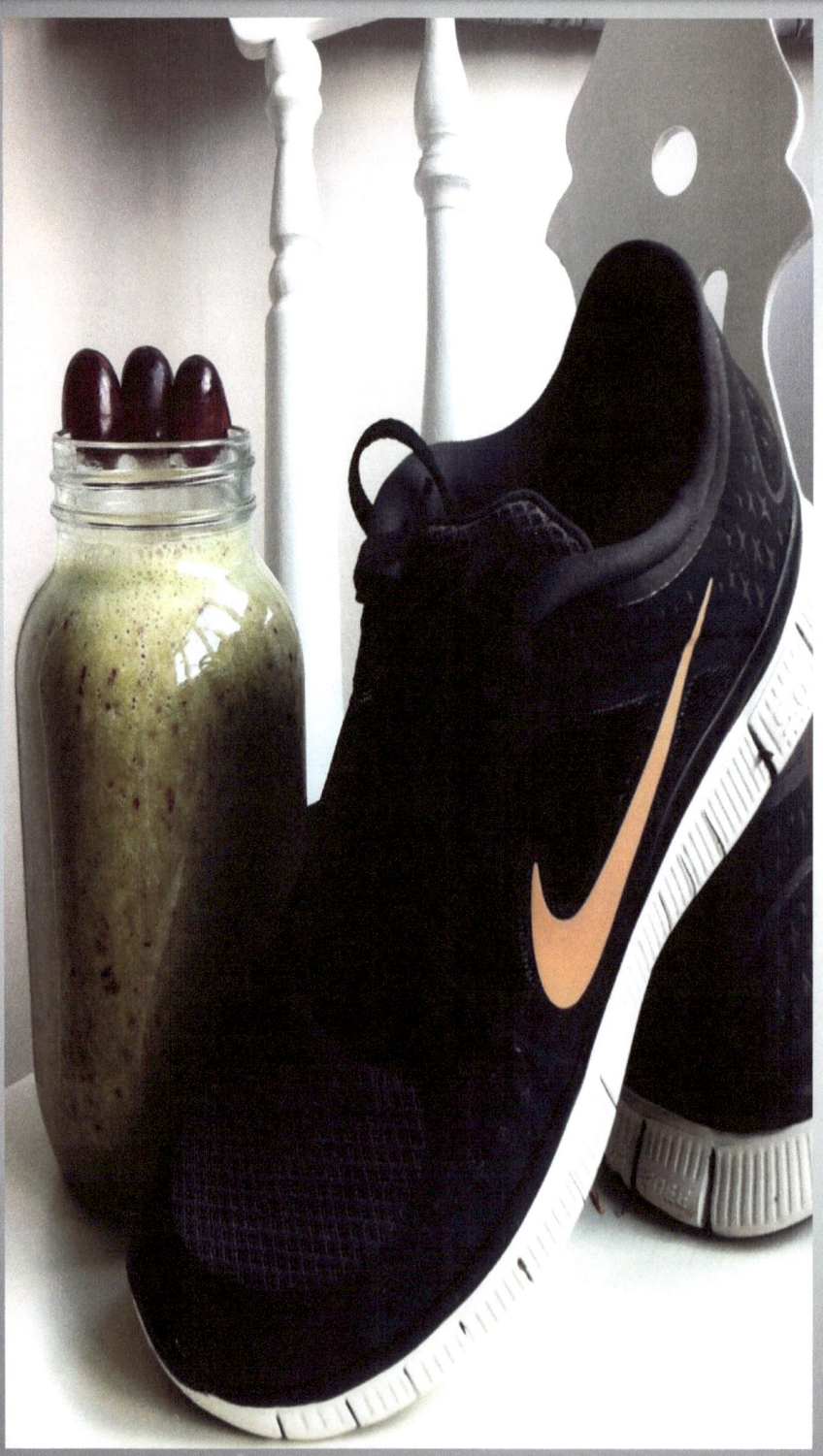

- bananas
- red grapes
- water

This is a beautiful combination, super sweet and yummy. Great as a post workout drink/snack or a meal depending on how big you like your smoothies. I make it BIG, so it serves as my breakfast post-run, e.g.

A Classic

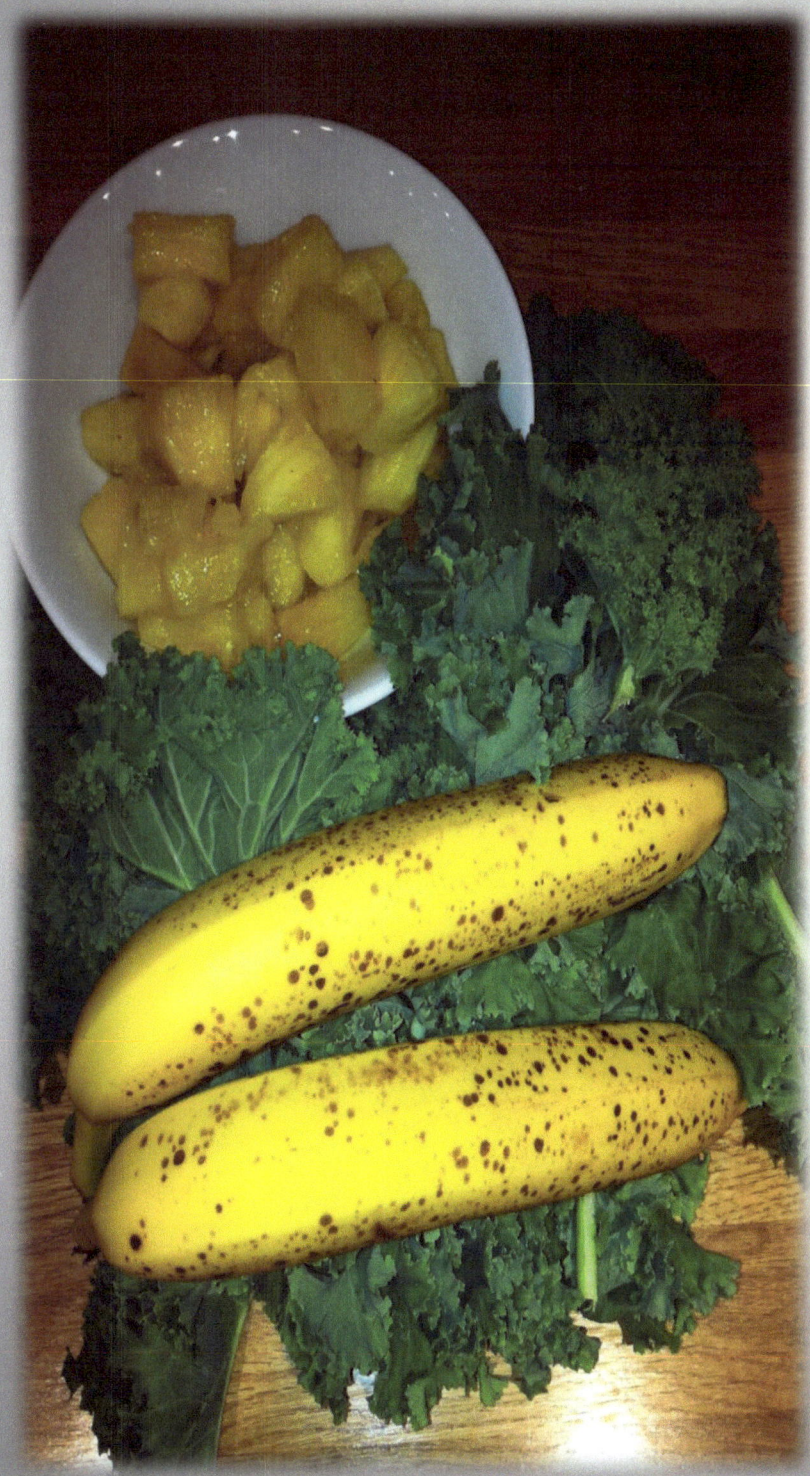

- bananas
- kale (can replace with spinach)
- pineapple
- water

This is my favourite classic green smoothie. Super simple. Just blend all ingredients together.

Green Berry Smoothie

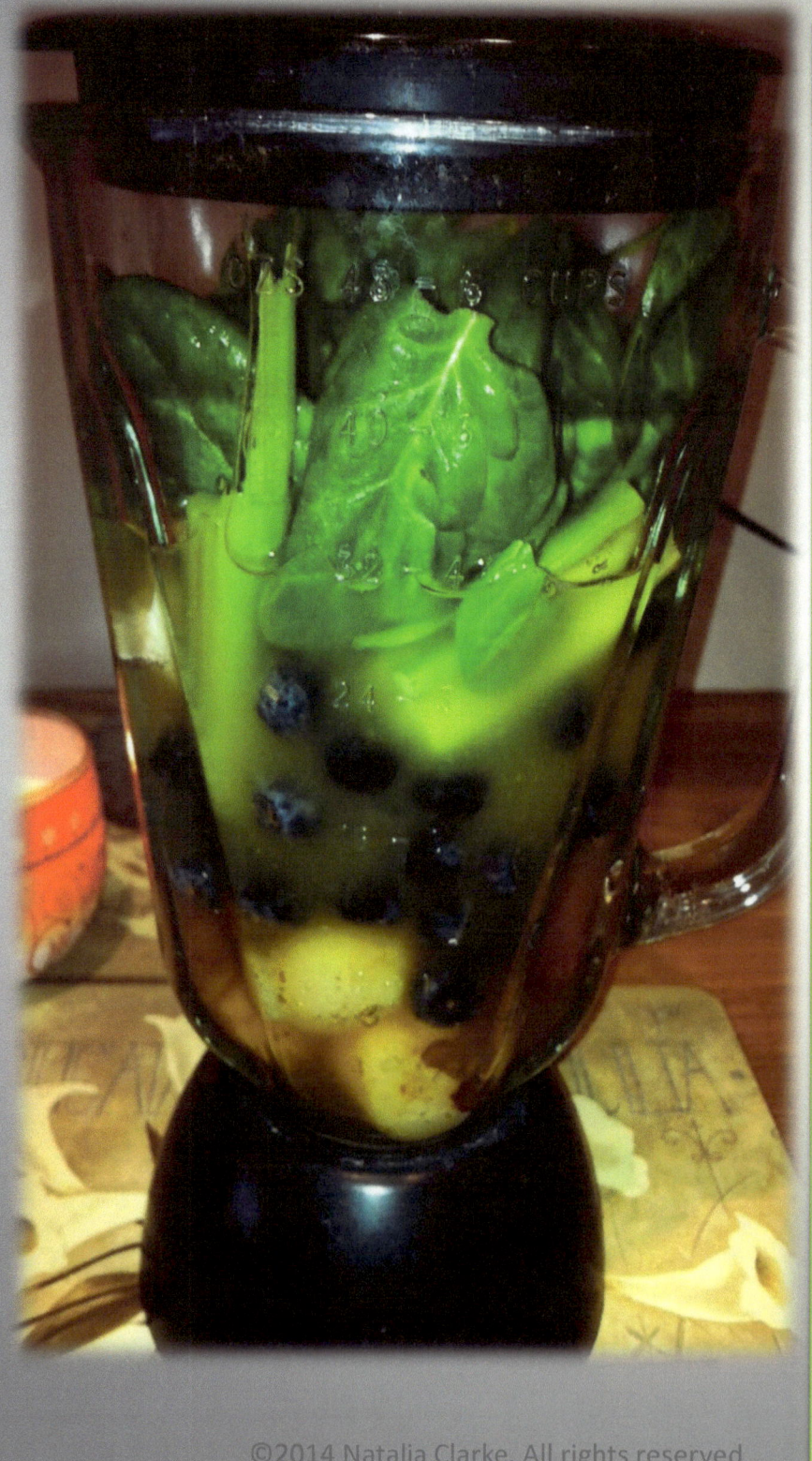

- bananas
- celery
- spinach
- blueberries
- water (pineapple juice)

Blend together and enjoy

28

Raw Juices

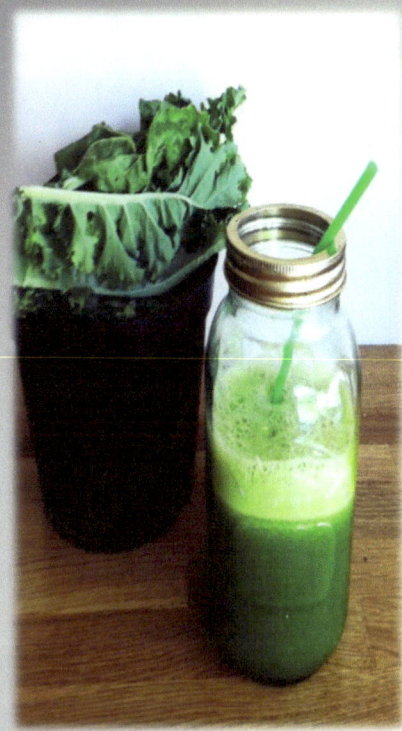
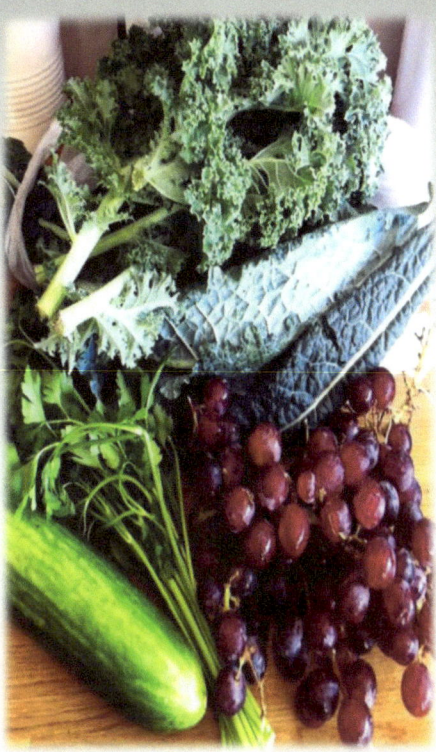
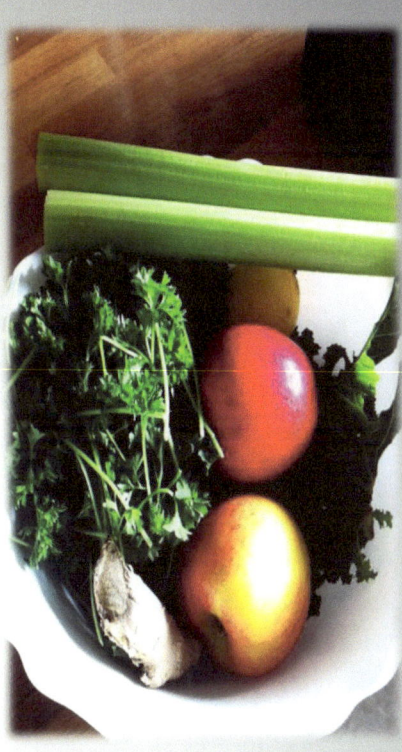
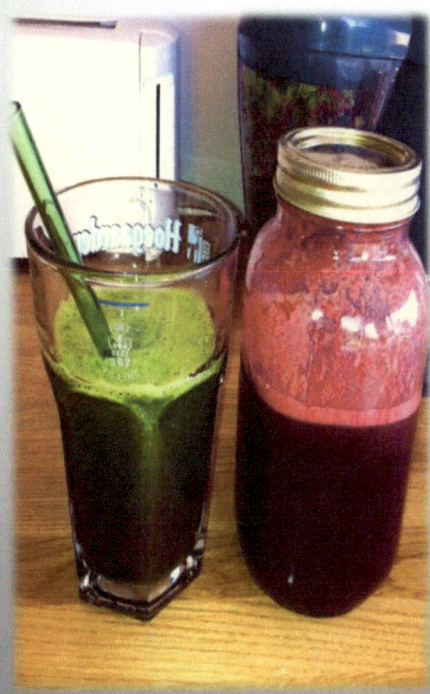
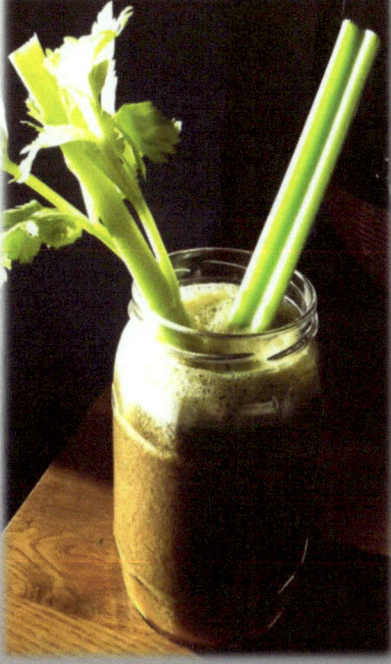

Juices ingredients

GREENS & HERBS	FRUIT	OTHER
Celery Cucumber Kale Spinach Spring greens Chard Beets' ends Parsley Mint Lettuce Broccoli Courgette	For sweetness please add: Apples Carrots Grapes (red grapes cut through bitterness well) Beetroot	Broccoli Courgette Cucumber Lemon Orange Ginger

Fruit Meals & Sweets

These are all LOW-fat FRUIT based MEALS (apart from my Lemon balls and brownies, which I usually only make once a year or so). Simple, nutritious AND delicious. Most of them are mono-meals (one fruit at a time), just cut up, peel, tear and devour. Eat as much as you want until fully satisfied.

I would normally have a mono-meal or a mixed fruit meal as a breakfast and lunch option. Remember to eat seasonally and only ripe fruit.

Mono-fruit Meals

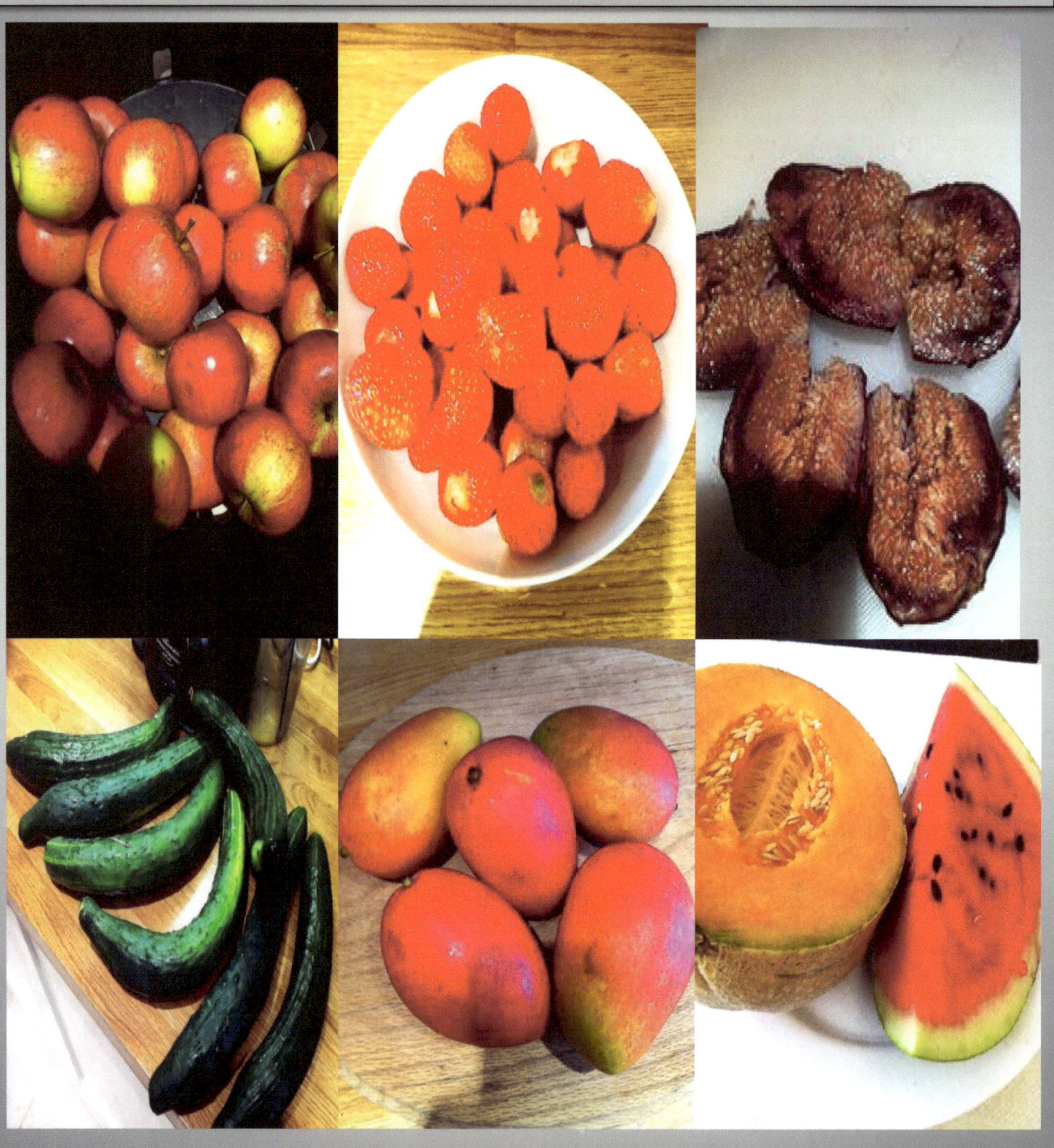

More mono-meals

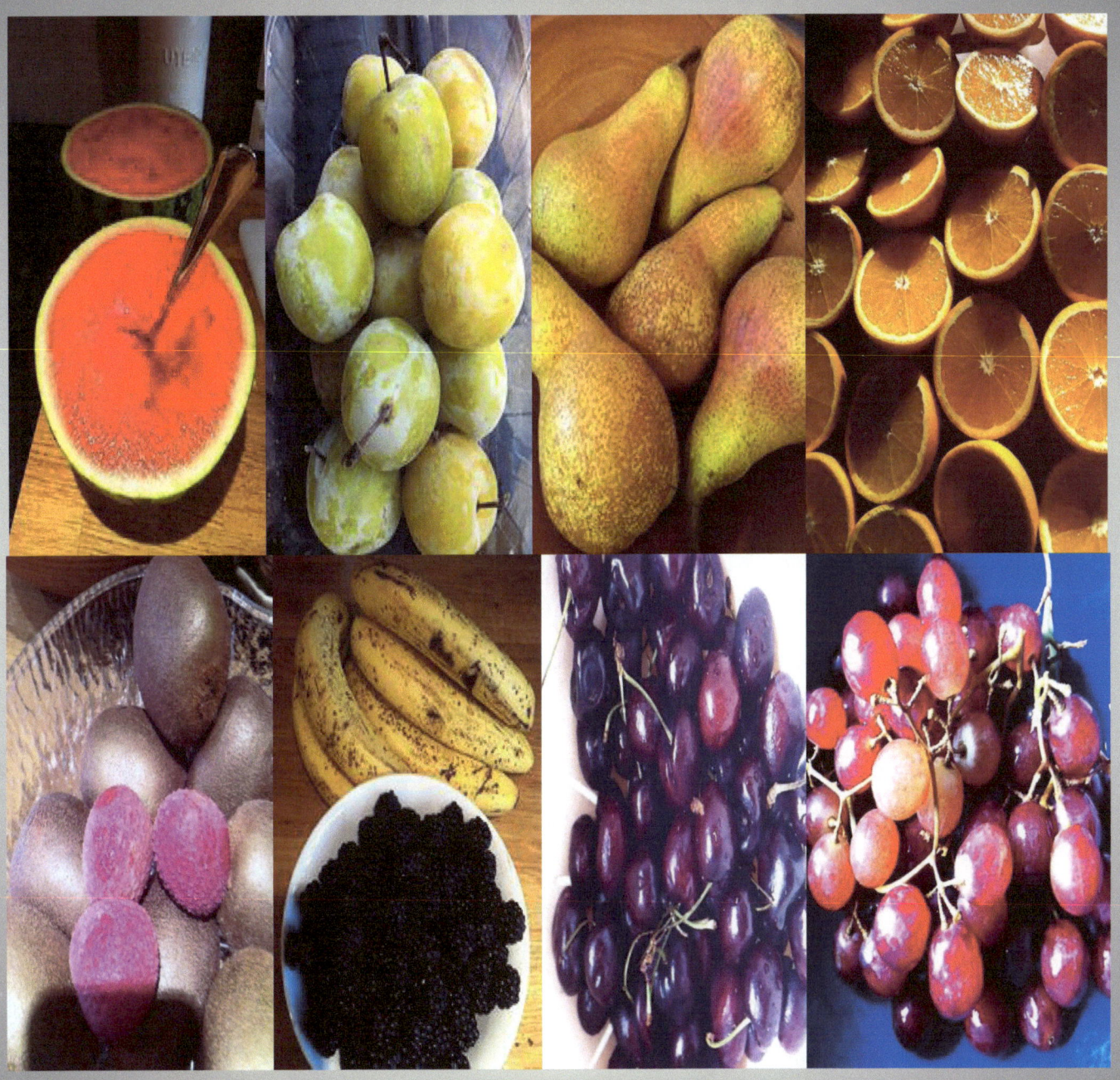

Mango & Blueberry Meal

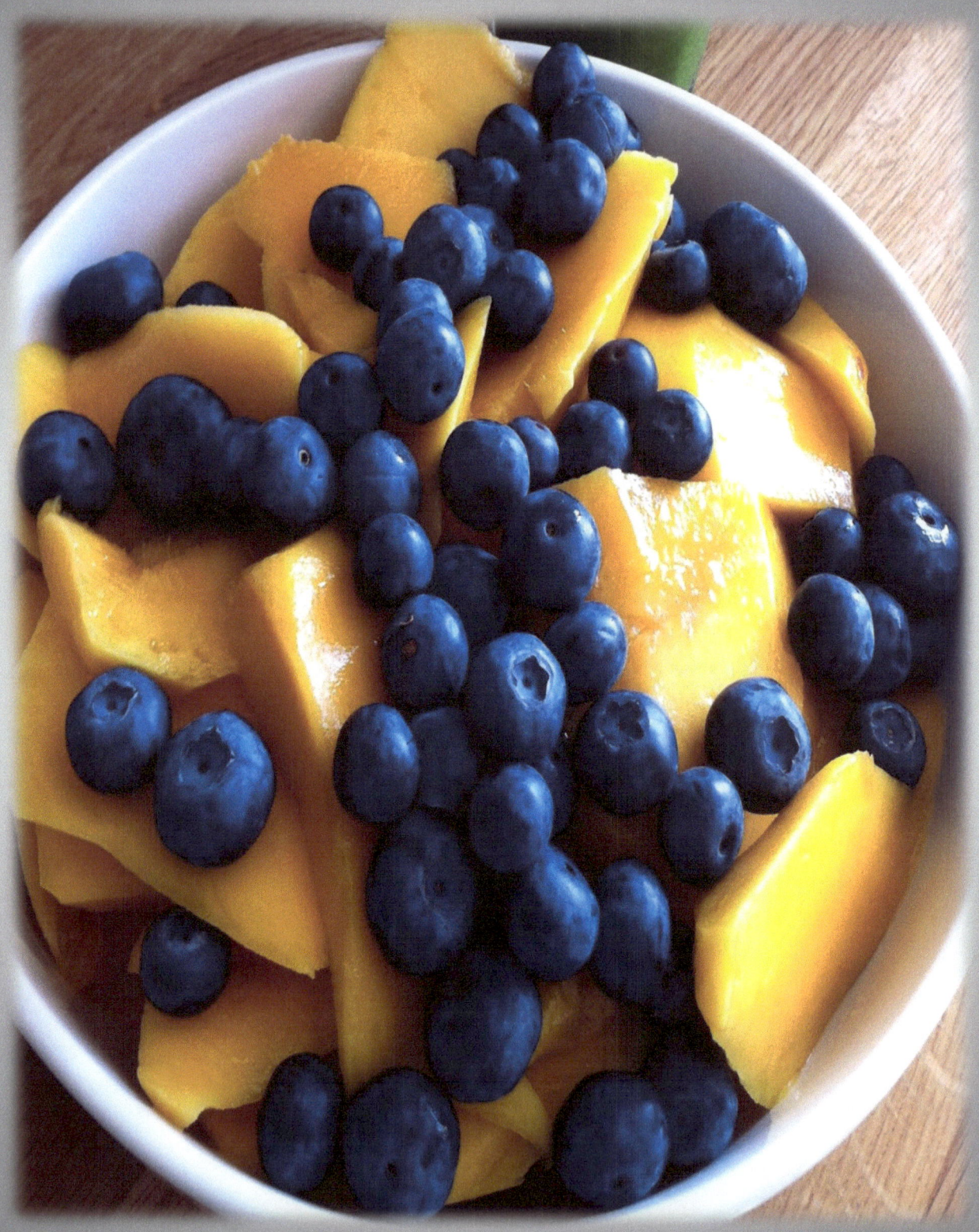

Papaya & Kiwi Meal

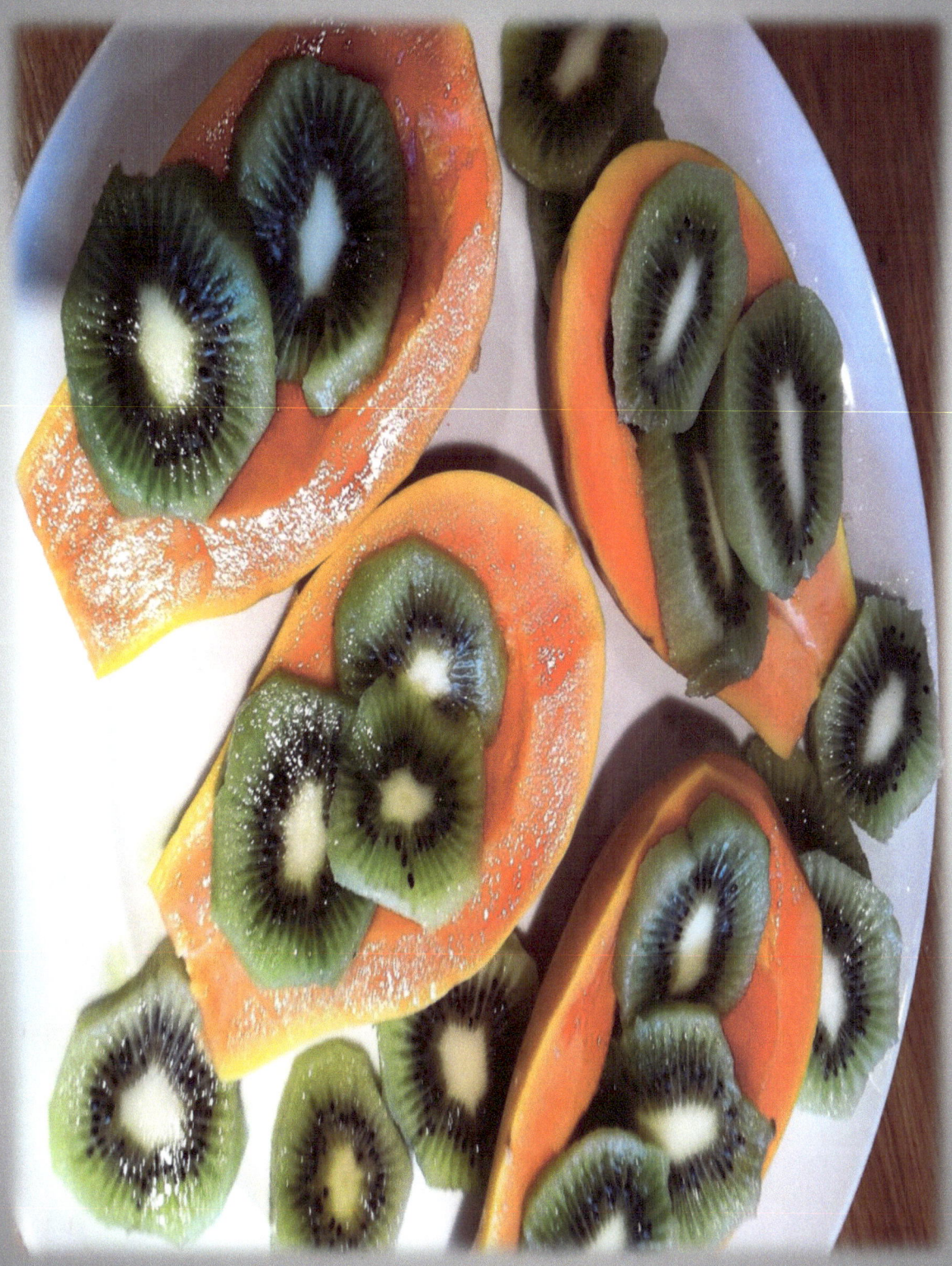

Pears & Raspberries Meal

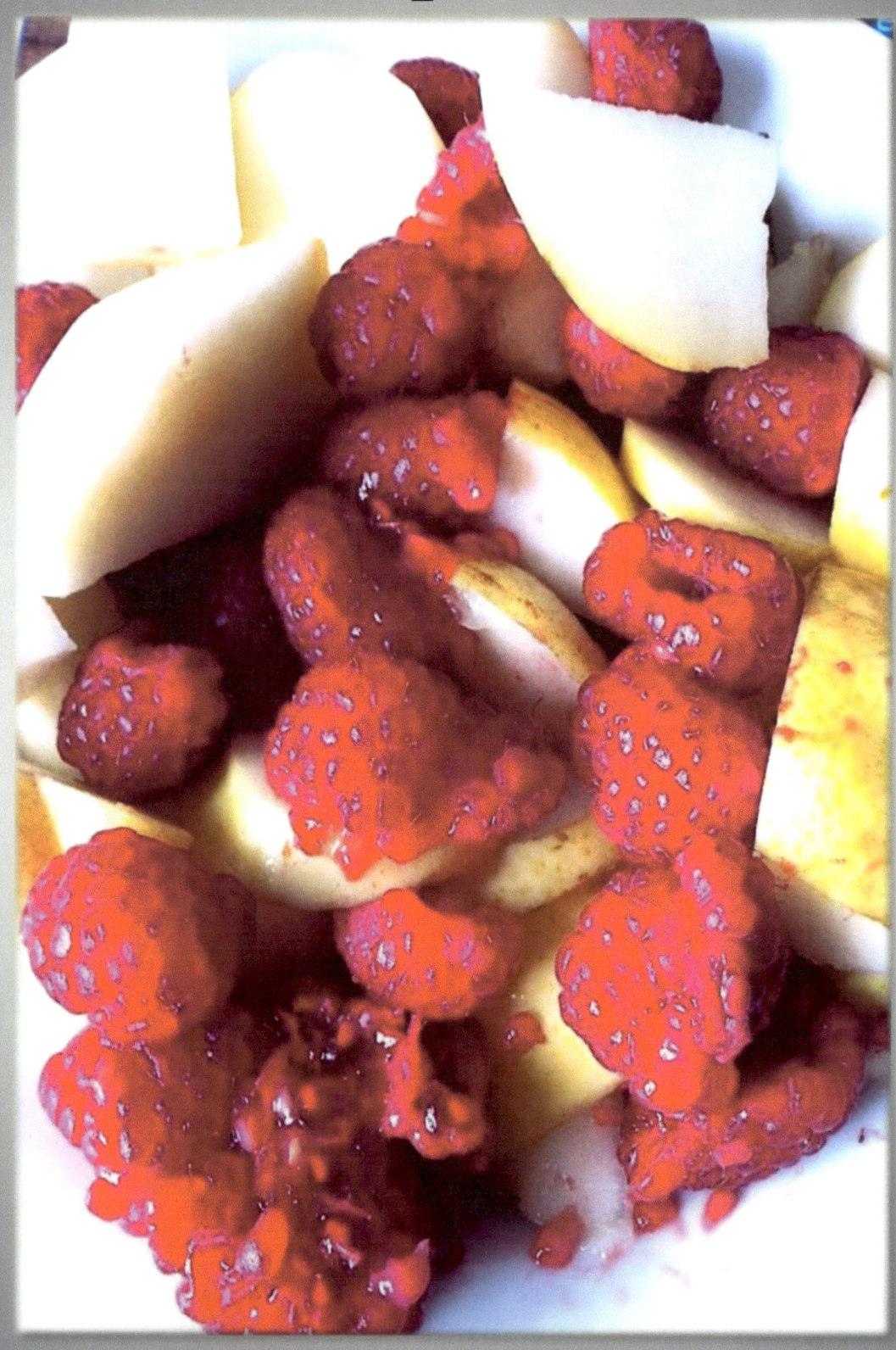

36

Mango with Raspberry Sauce

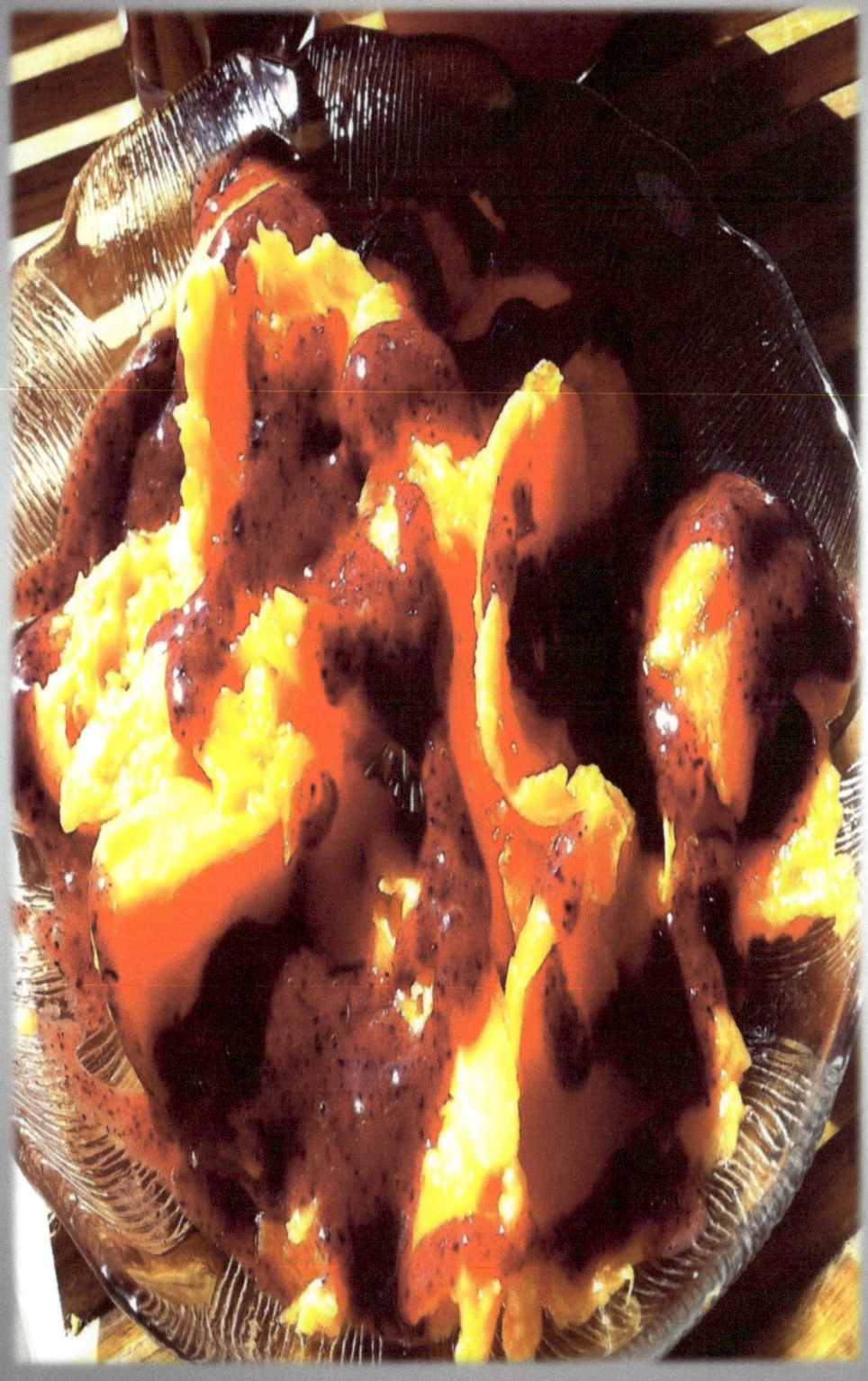

For raspberry sauce simply blend fresh raspberries

Bananas with Strawberry Sauce

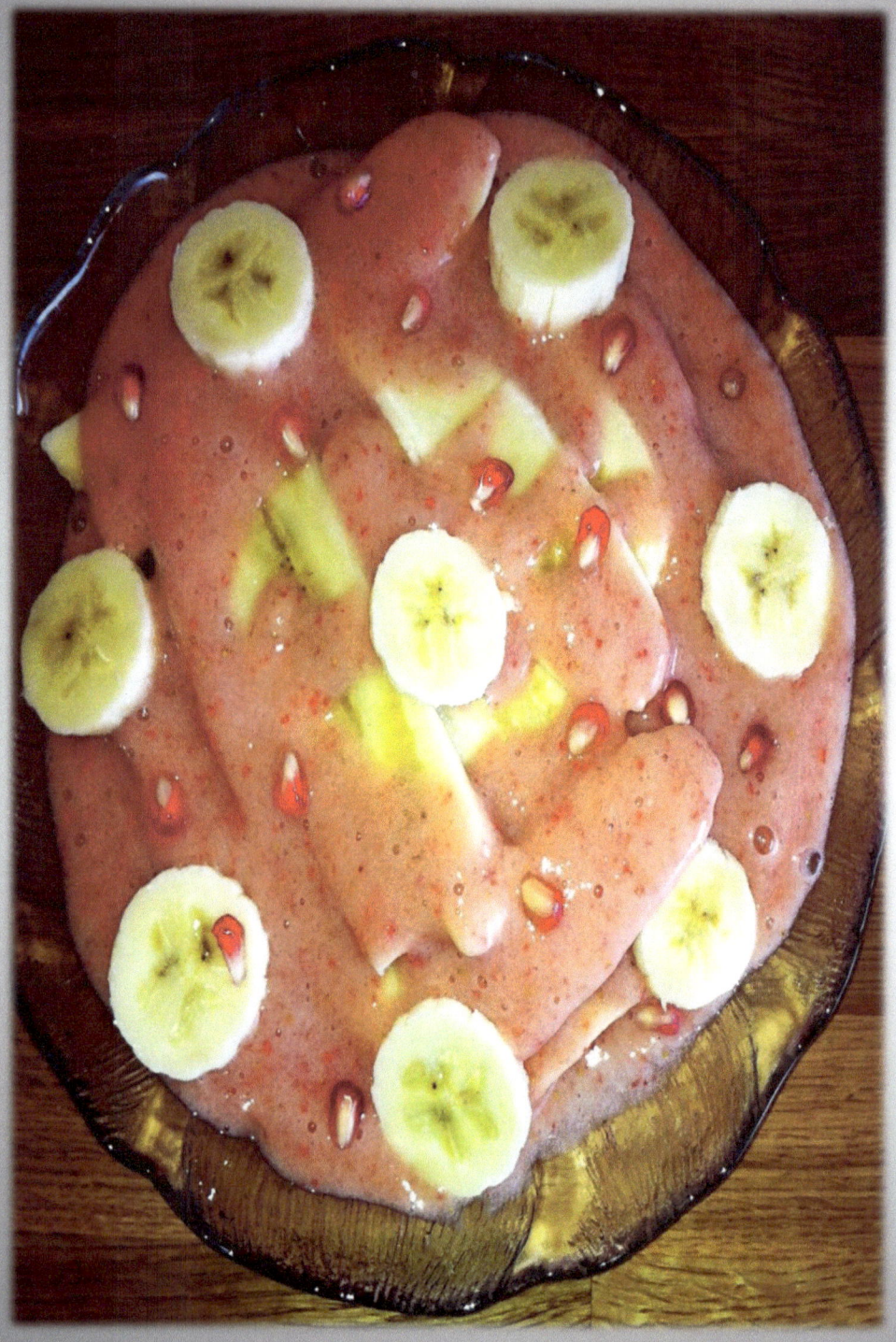

For the sauce just blend fresh strawberries. Can be done with any berries of your choice

38

Meal in a Jar

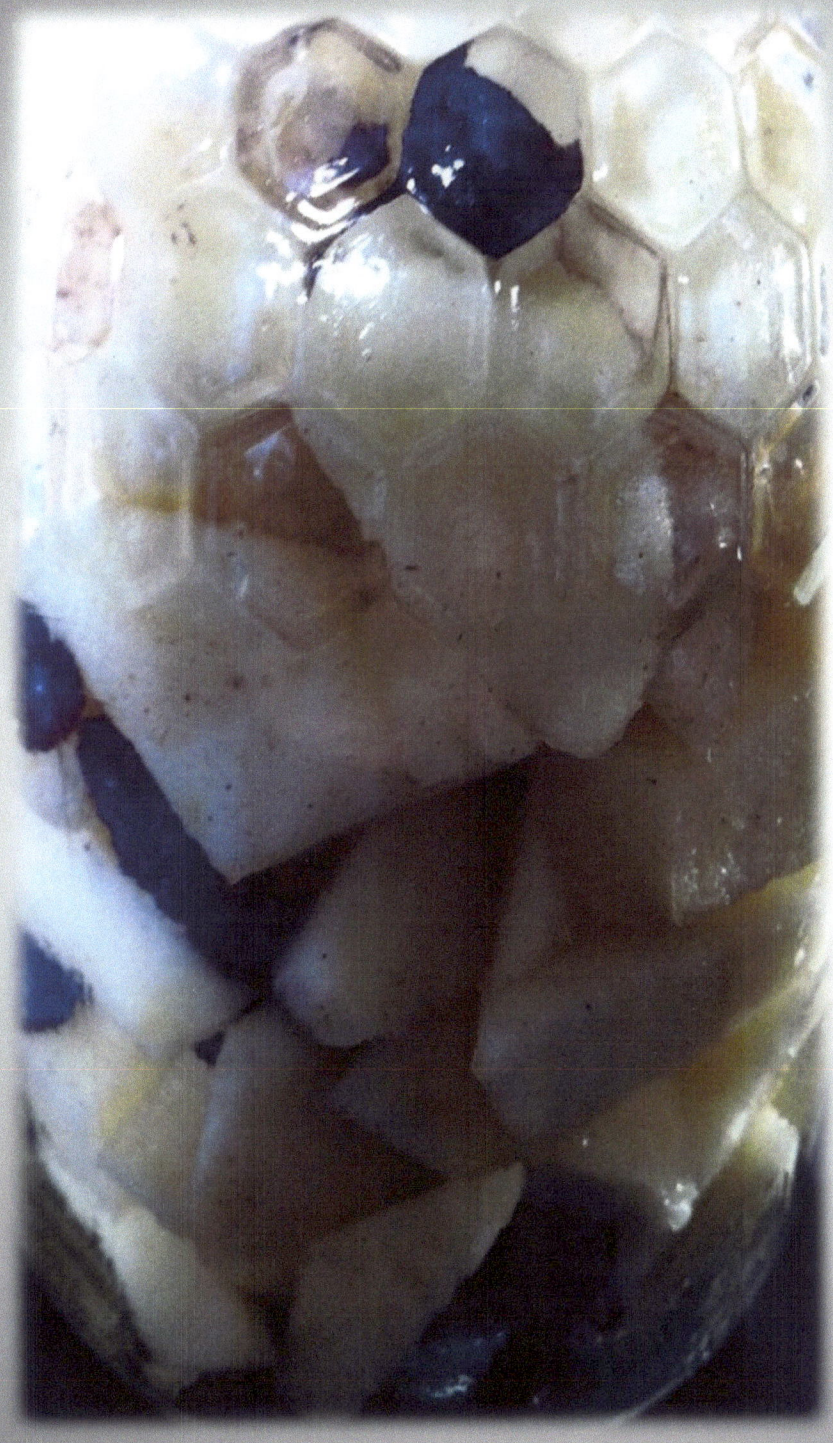

- apples
- raisins
- bananas
- coconut water
- cinnamon

Nice and portable meal.

Fruit Ice-cream

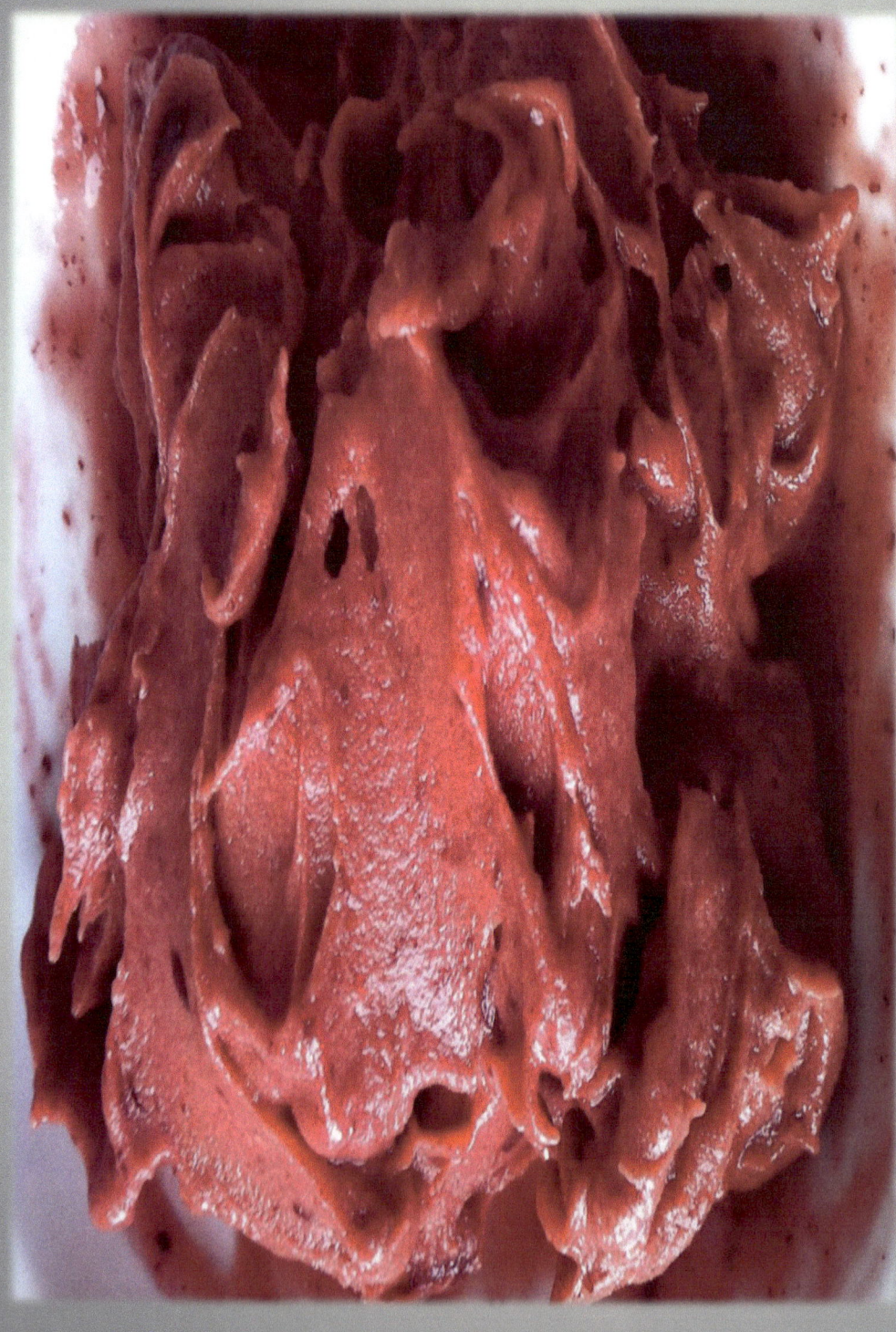

- frozen bananas
- frozen cherries
- a touch of water

Blend in a high-speed blender like Vitamix, e.g. And enjoy straight away. Flavours can be varied – just replace cherries with strawberry, blueberry, pineapple or mango blend with frozen bananas as a base. Delicious!

40

Banana Ice-cream

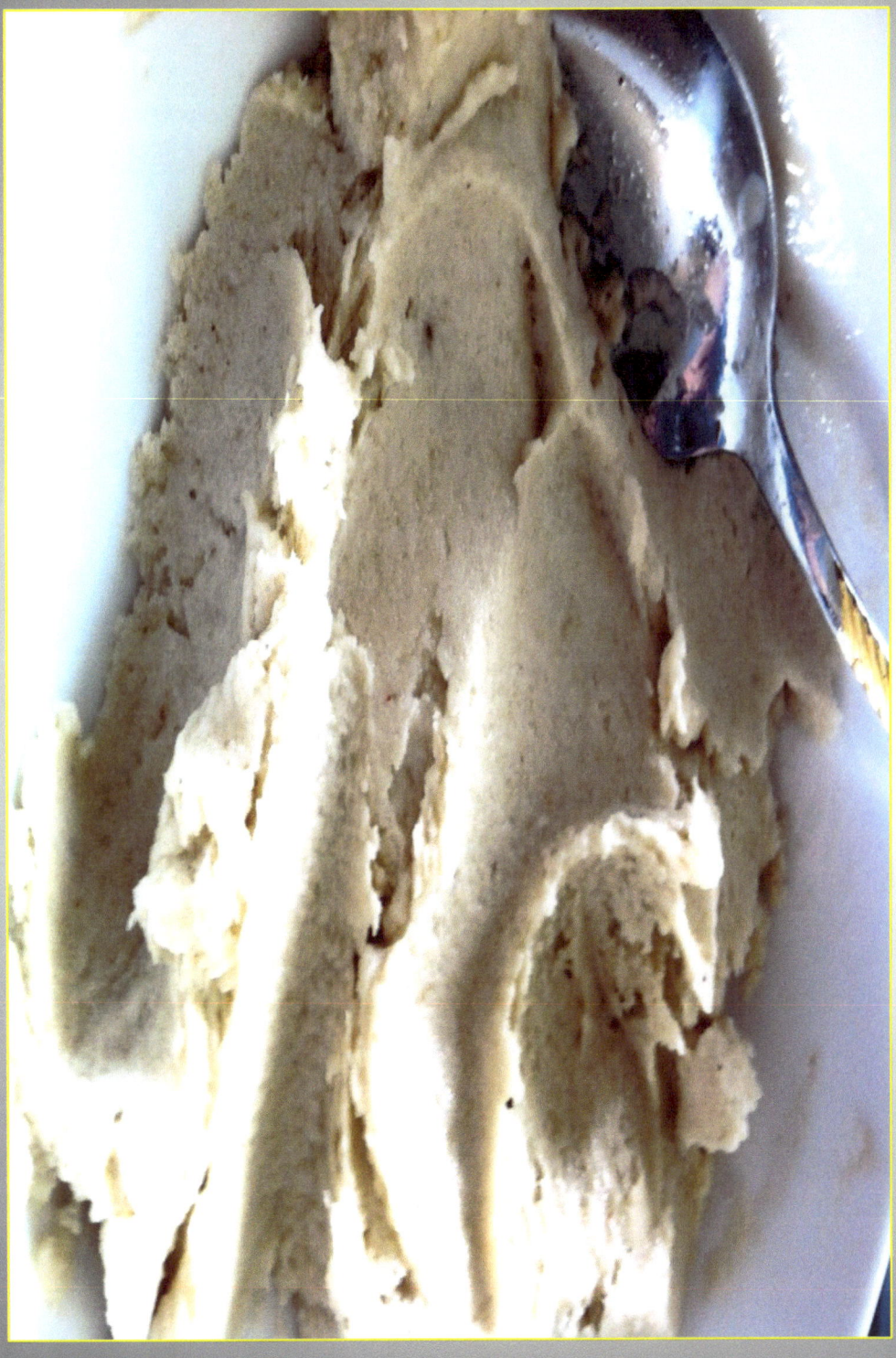

• frozen bananas
• a touch of water

Possibilities with flavours are endless with this meal. Use frozen bananas as a base and add peppermint tea, vanilla, dates chunks, raw choc chips, carob powder (for chocolate taste), peanut butter. Be inventive!

Strawberry Ice-cream with date sauce

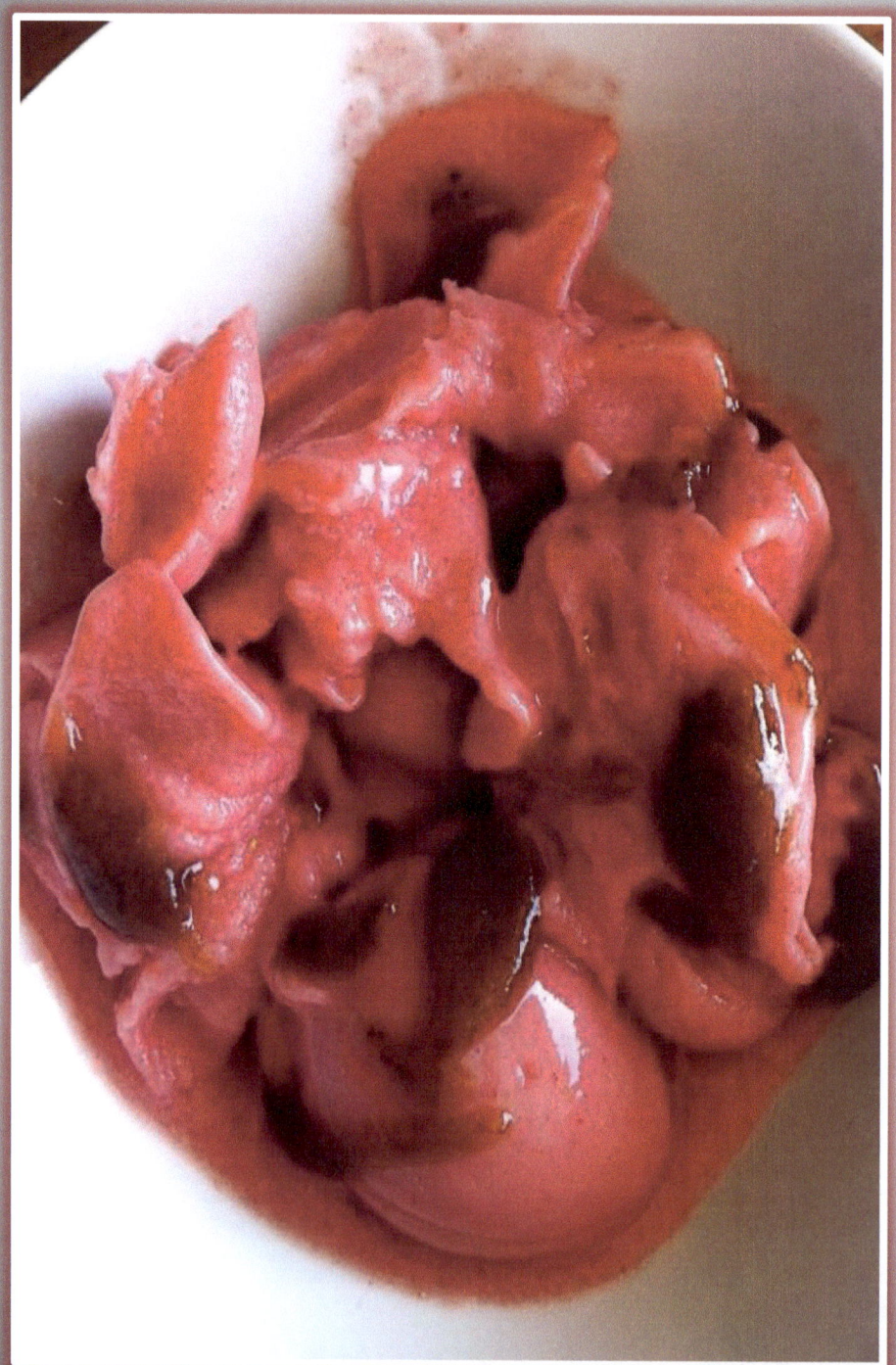

- a touch of water
- frozen bananas
- frozen strawberries
- dates soaked blended (sauce)

Blend bananas and strawberries in a high speed blender. Pour dates sauce over

Raw 'eggs'

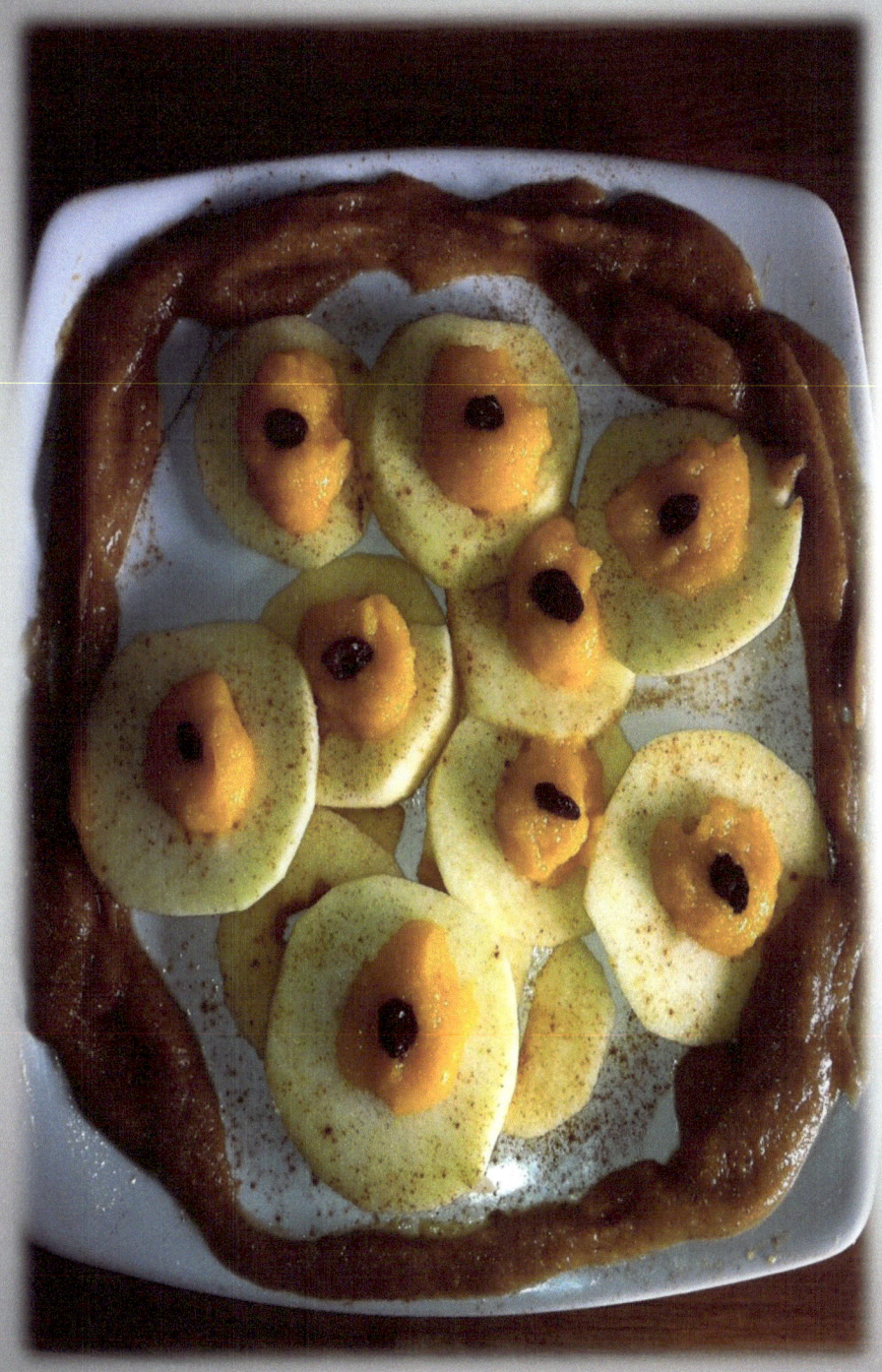

- apples
- raisins
- dates
- apricots
- lemon juice

Cut apples into rings. Yellow sauce (apricots blended with water); brown sauce (dates blended with water and apricots). Can add a touch of lemon juice to both sauces if desired

Apple Pudding

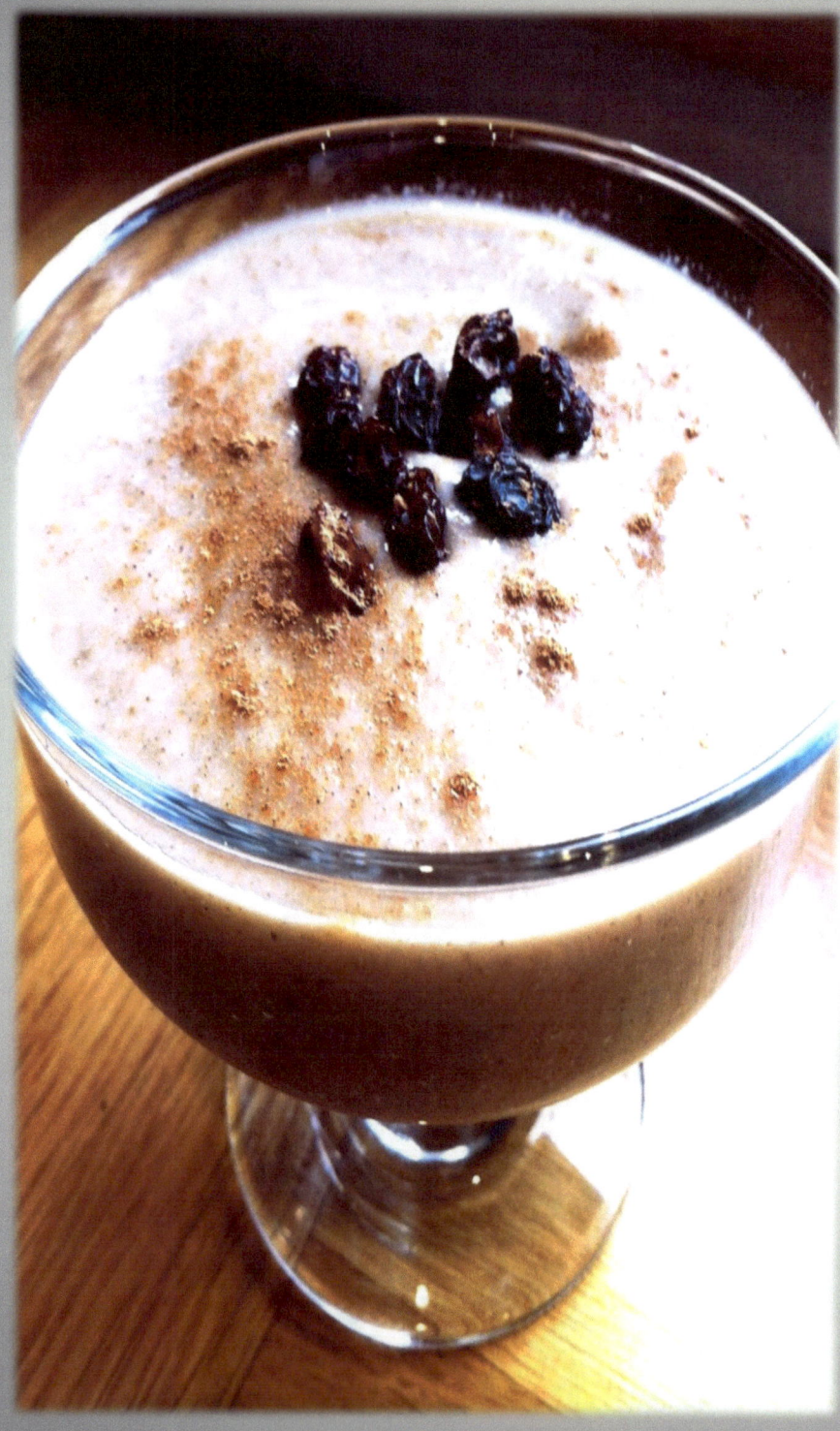

- apples
- bananas
- cinnamon
- chia seeds (soak for 10 mins till it becomes jelly-like)

Mix all together once chia seeds are jellified and enjoy

Satsumas with Sauce

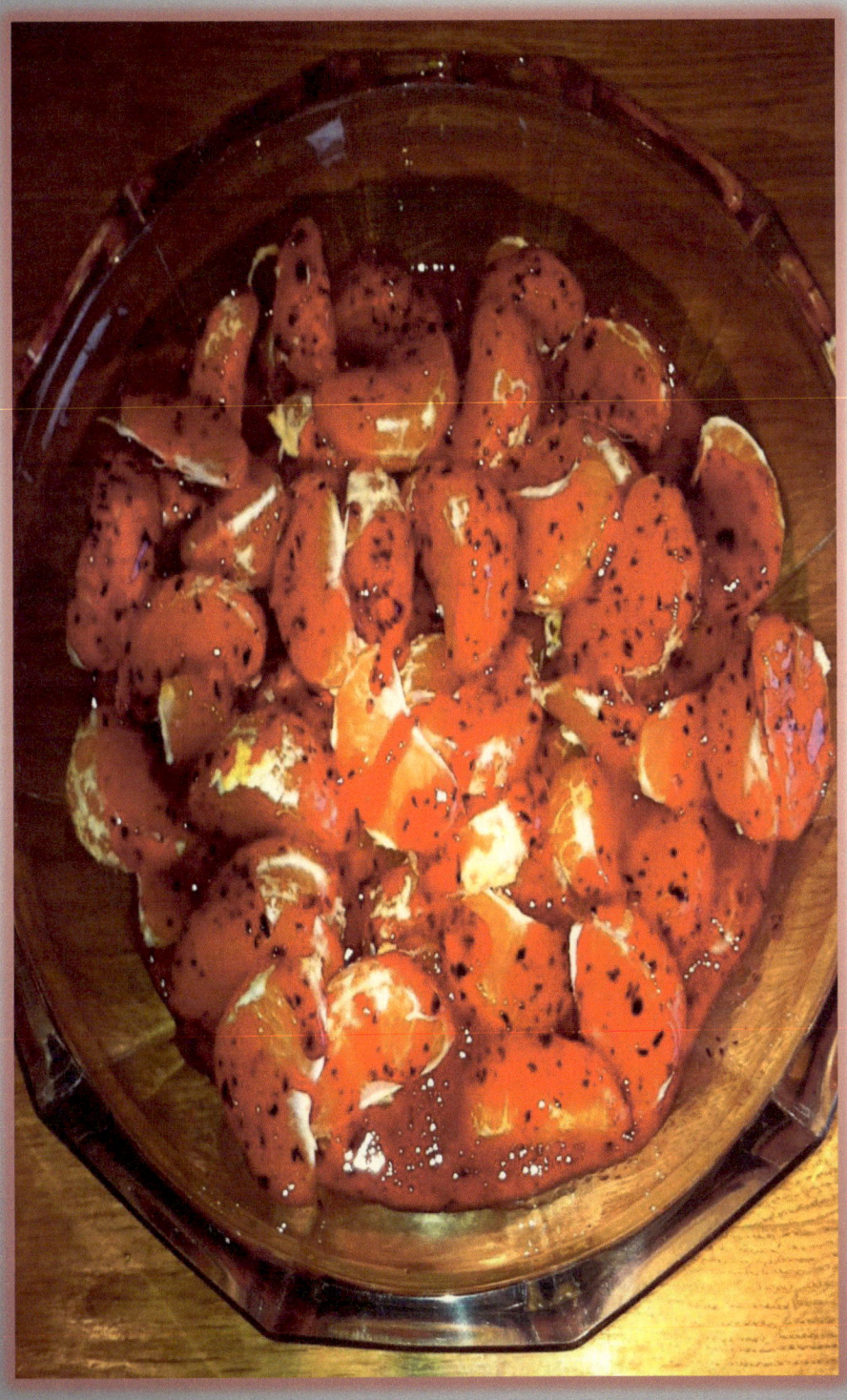

for the sauce just blend either fresh raspberries or blueberries and enjoy

45

Pears with Raspberry Sauce

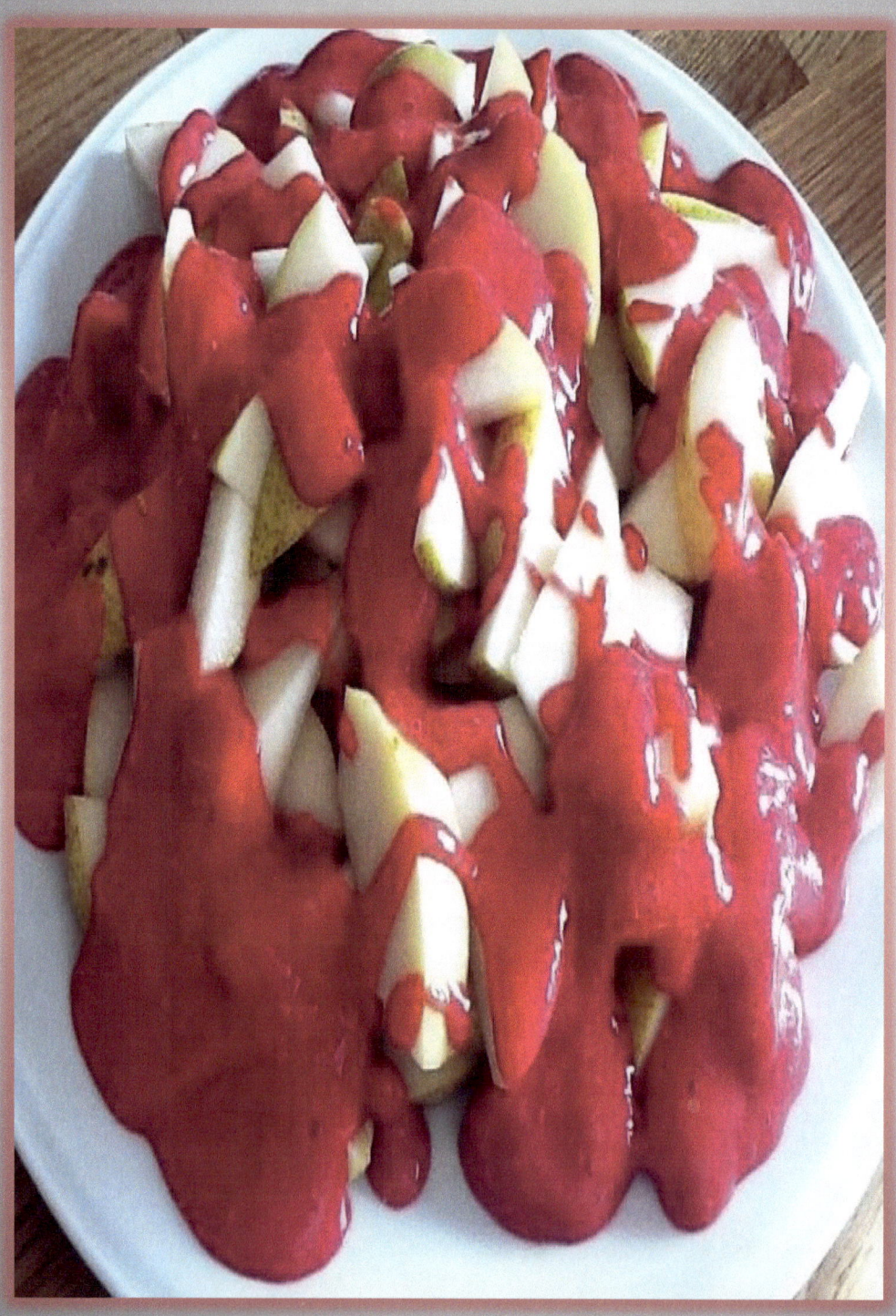

for the sauce just blend fresh raspberries

46

Lemon Balls

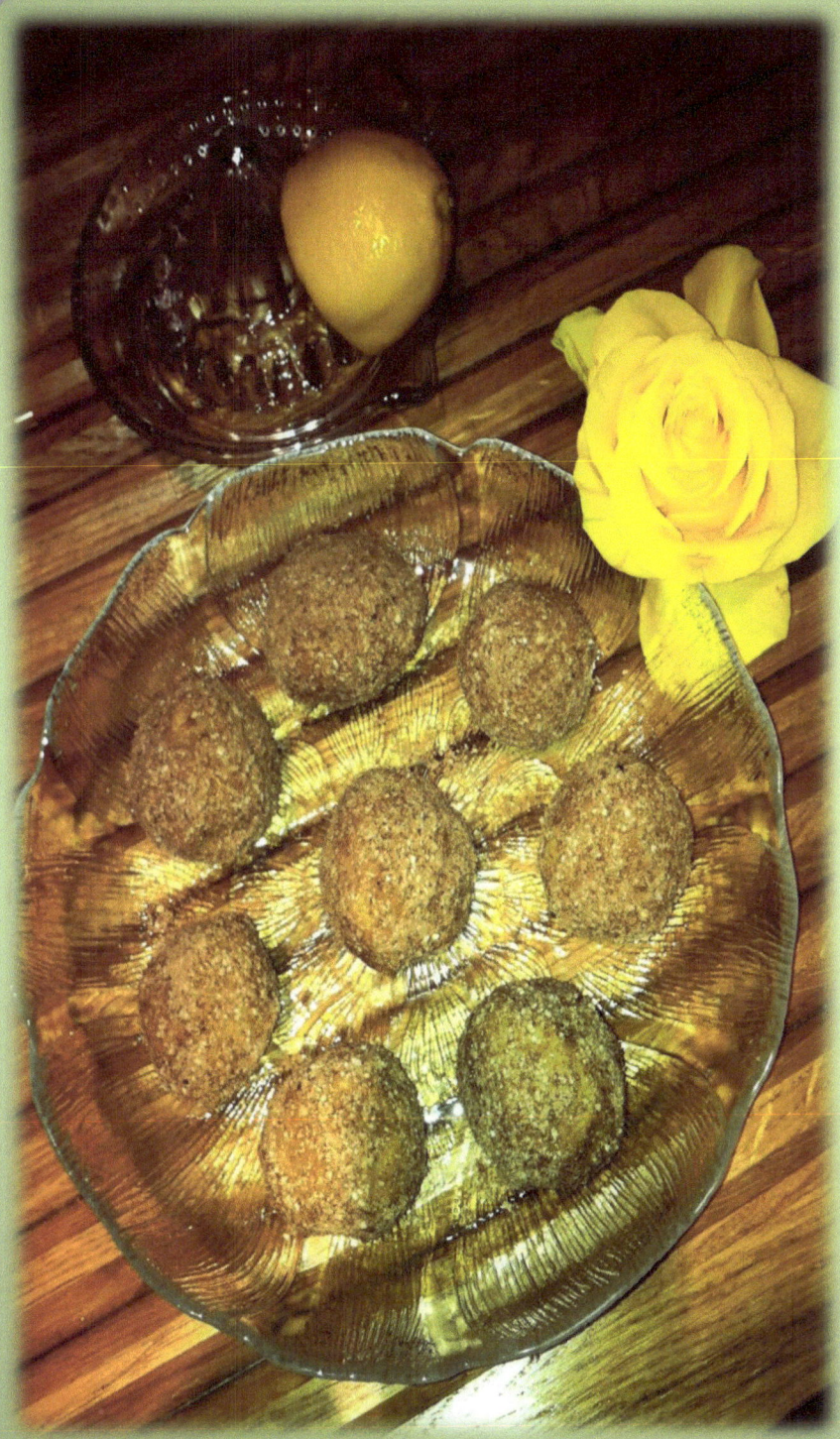

- walnuts/almonds
- lemon juice
- lemon zest
- dates (soft)
- vanilla
- almond powder (almonds powdered in a food processor)
- salt (optional)

Mix everything together to your desired consistency and taste (as much or as little lemon as you want and the same with dates depending on how sweet you want it) and put in the fridge for an hour. Roll into balls in almond powder

47

Raw Brownies

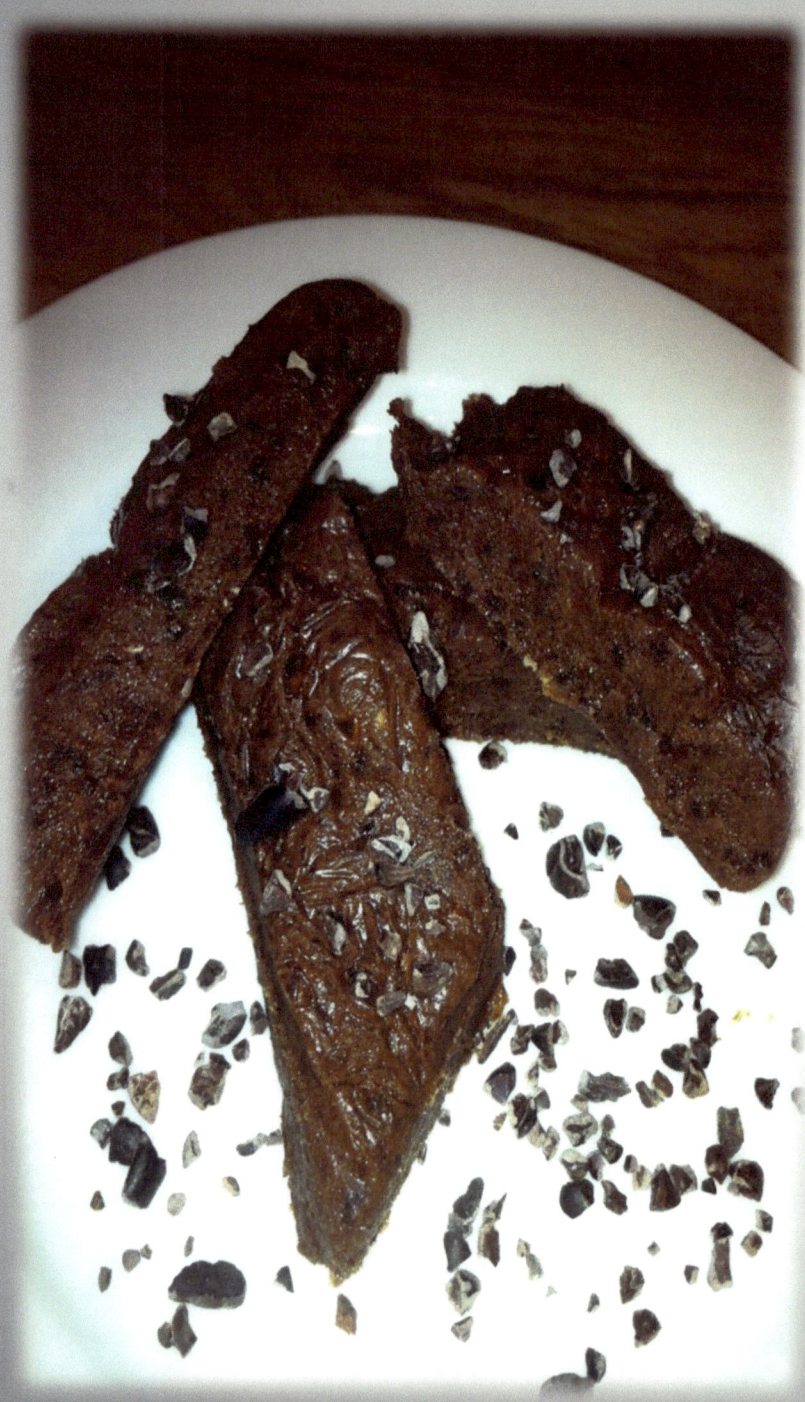

- coconut oil
- raw choc chips
- dates
- lemon juice
- carob powder
- walnuts/almonds

Mix everything together to your desired consistency and put in a freezer. Once it solidifies, cut into brownie pieces

48

Apple Soup

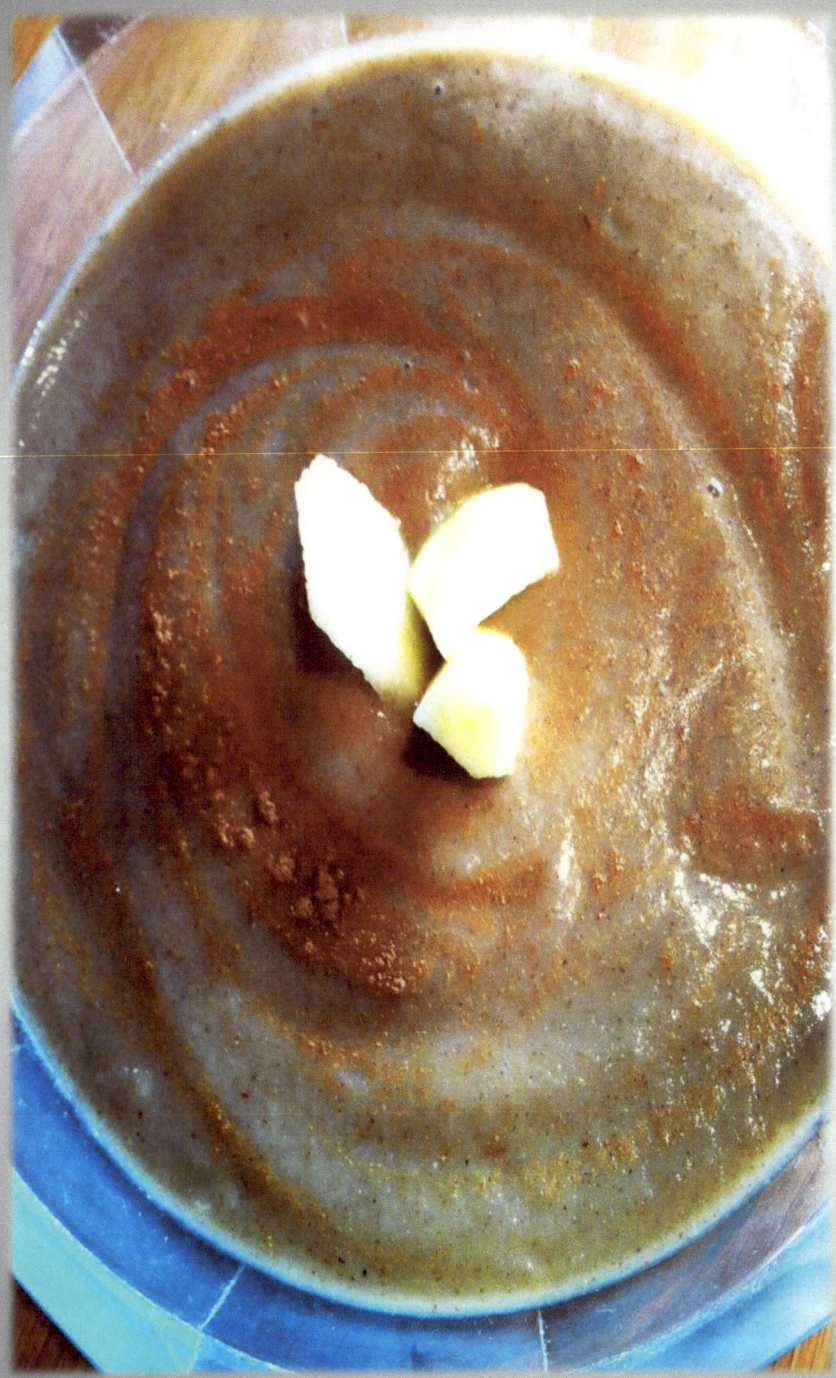

- 3 to 4 apples
- frozen banana
- carob powder (optional)
- cinnamon
- vanilla essence

Blend all together till smooth

49

Chia Pudding

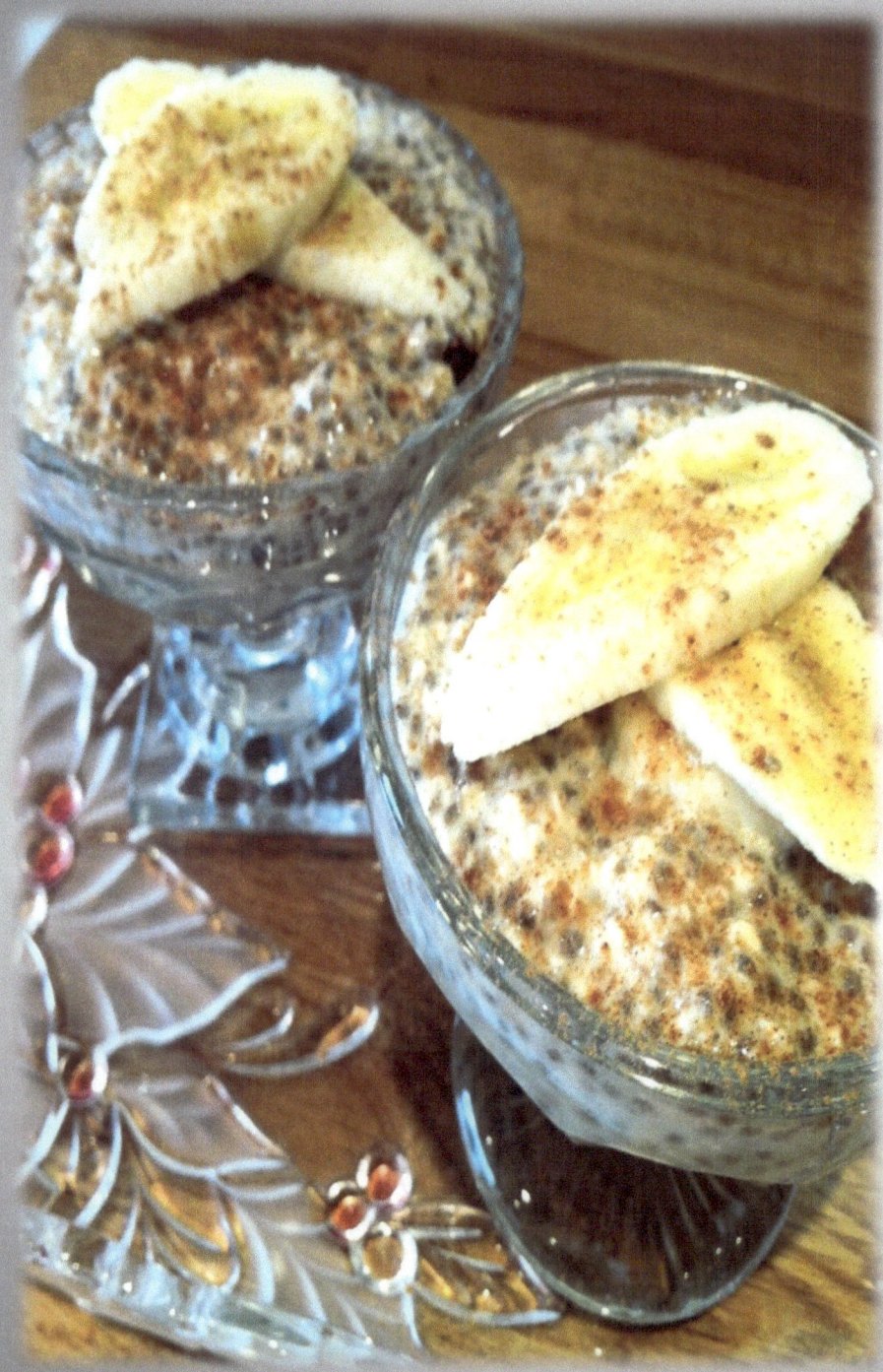

- chia seeds
- oats
- raisins
- banana sliced
- carob powder
- almond milk
(can also add
pineapple juice)
Put all ingredients in
a jar and fill up with
almond milk and
leave overnight. Eat
for breakfast the next
day. Super filling,
Omega 3 and protein
rich meal

50

Evening Meals

Here I include savoury evening meals of salads, raw soups, snacks and sauces. To all of these dishes you can add nuts/seeds/avocado/olives for fats, if you like. I prefer low-fat meals. These meals' ingredients can easily be mixed and swapped depending on your taste preferences. Have fun!

Raw pasta with sauce

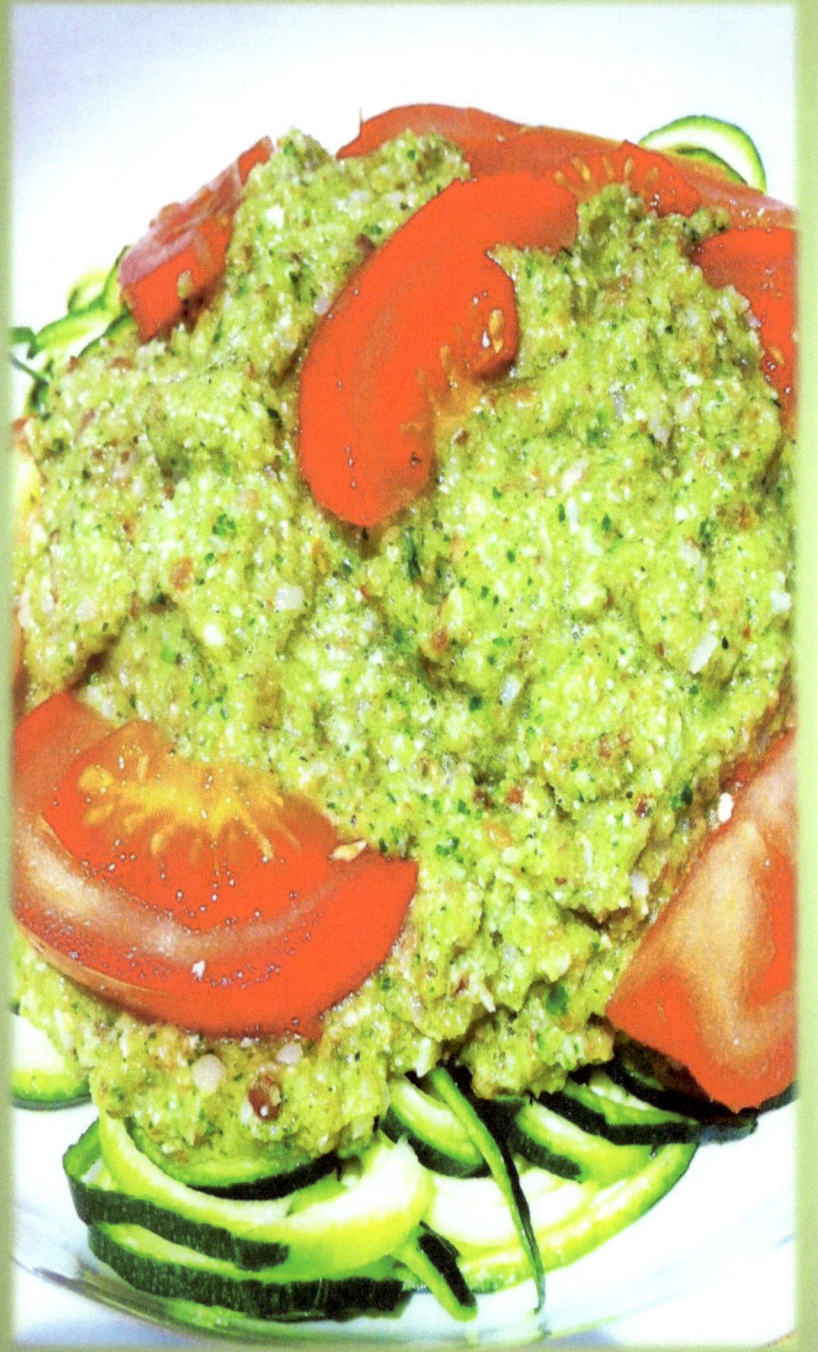

For the Sauce
- celery
- tomato
- garlic
- cucumber (peeled)
- mint & parsley (optional)
- red pepper
- courgette
- lemon juice

Make spaghetti noodles with a spiralizer from courgettes (zucchini). Mix all the ingredients above together and pour over. This dressing has a very fresh feel and will also be good over cauliflower rice (roughly blended raw cauliflower in a food processor)

Red Cabbage Meal

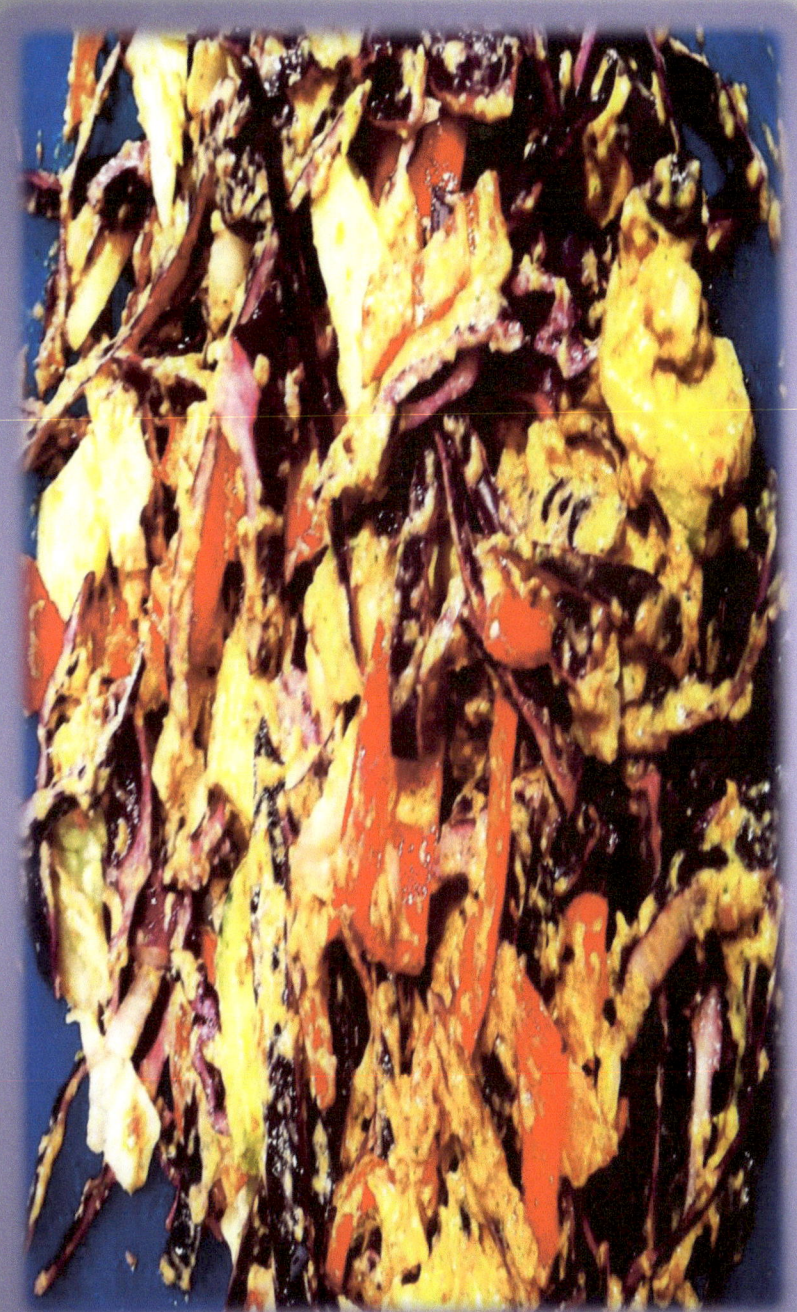

For the Dressing

- garlic
- sun dried tomatoes
- fresh tomatoes
- herbs of your choice
- olive oil (optional)
- ground nuts of your choice (optional)
- grapefruit juice

For the Salad

- shredded red cabbage
- onion (optional)
- cucumber chunks
- chopped red peppers

Romaine Salad with Beets sauce

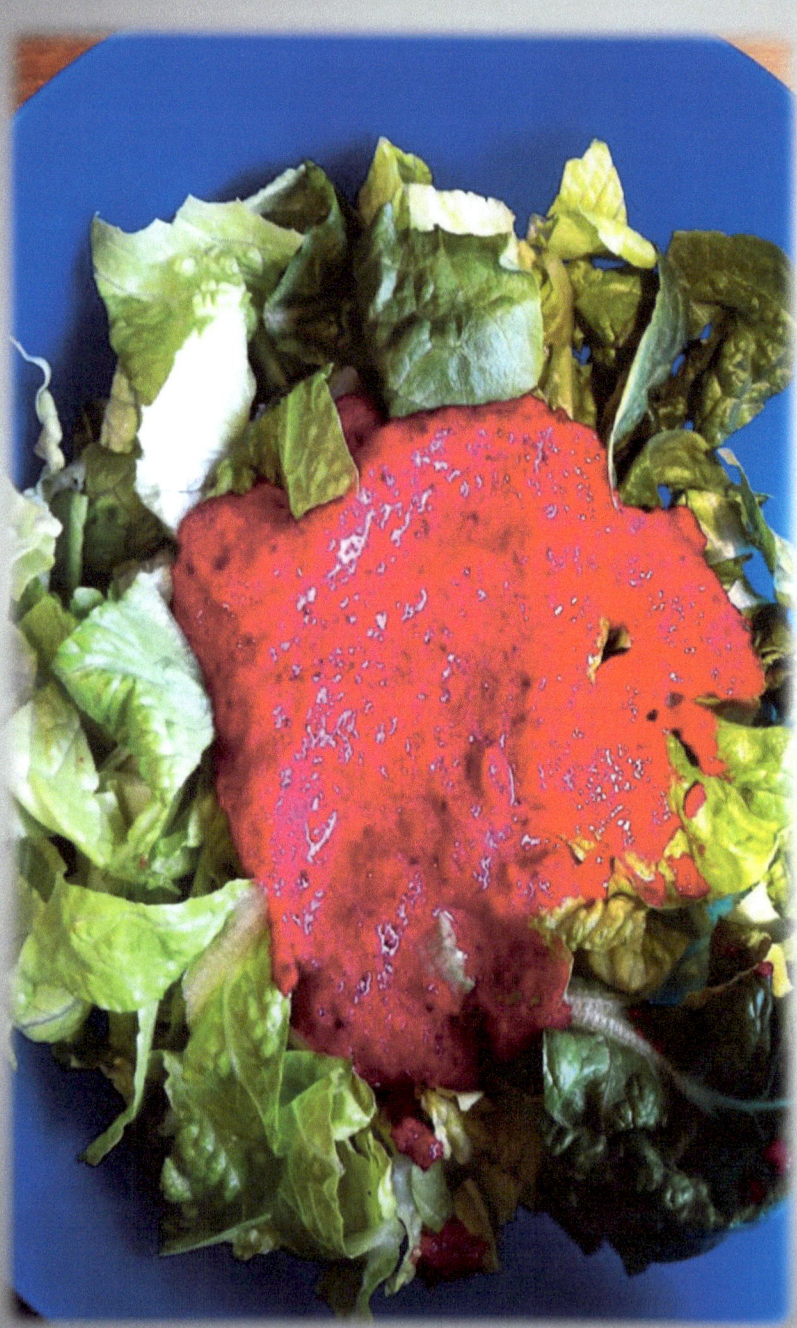

For the Dressing
- garlic
- fresh beet root
- fresh tomatoes
- walnuts (optional)

For the Salad
- Romaine lettuce
- spinach
- any other greens

Green Power Soup

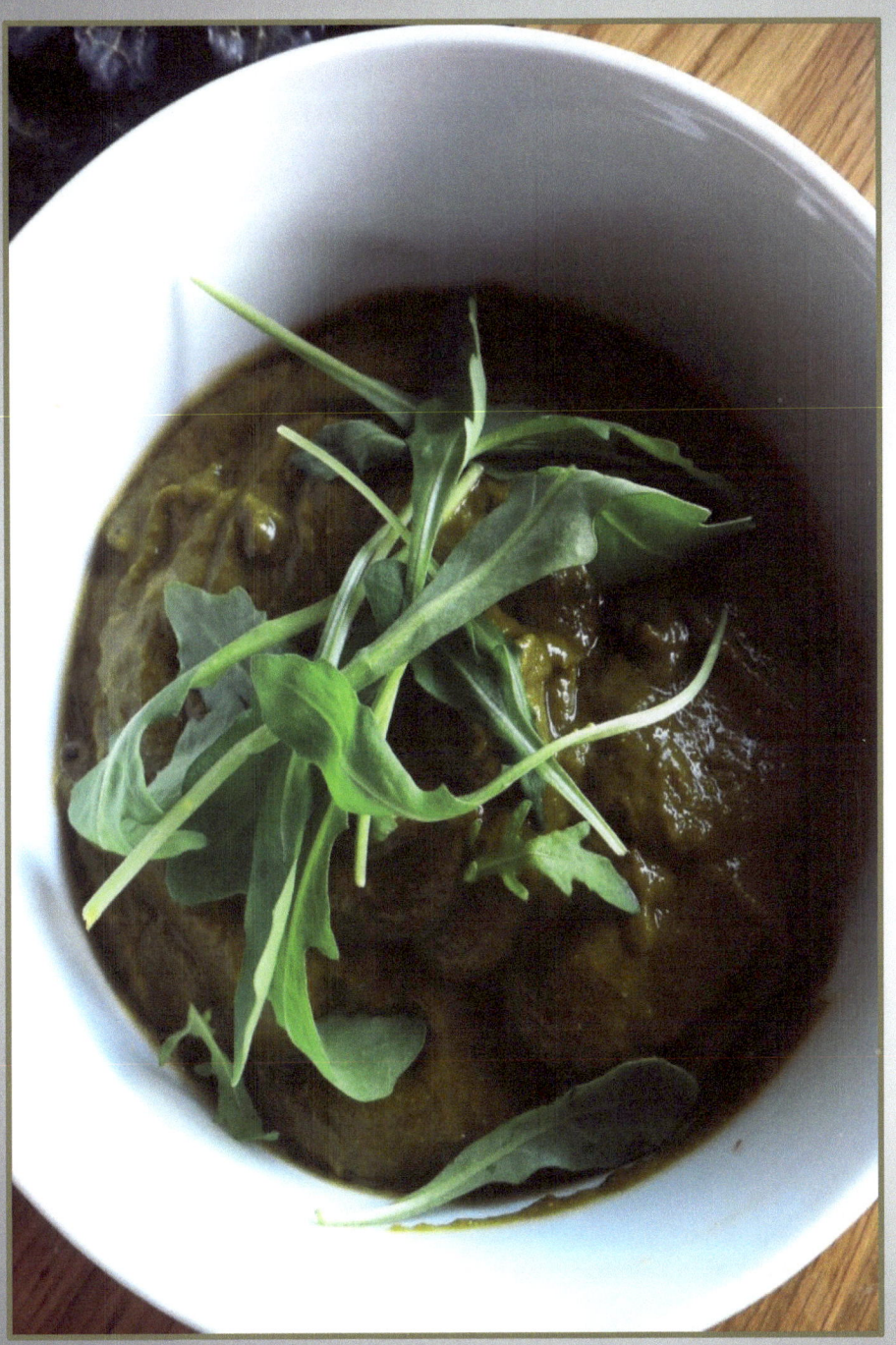

- kale
- spinach
- red pepper
- avocado
- garlic
- lemon juice

Blend all ingredients together and eat with a BIG spoon. Creamy, delicious & nutritious

55

Creamy Veggie Wraps

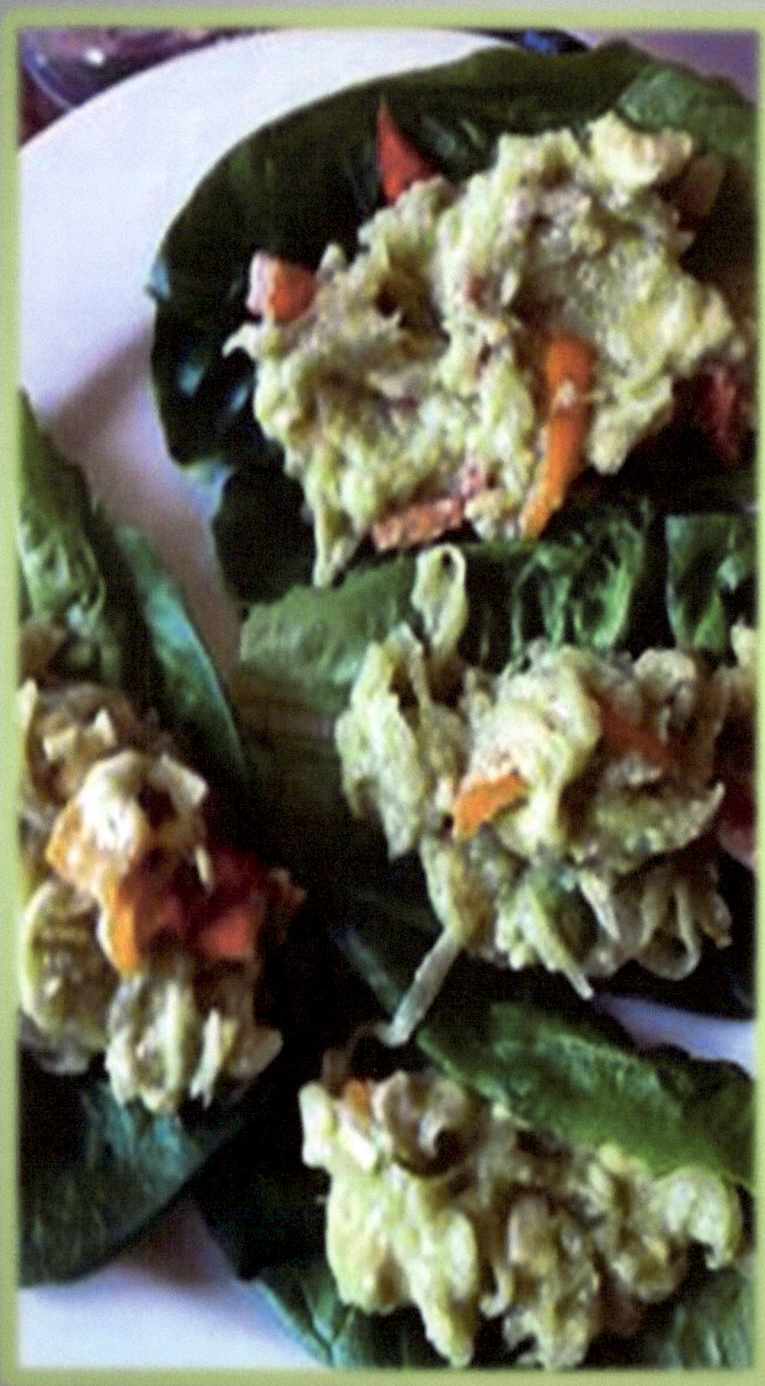

- grated peeled cucumbers
- almond butter
- avocado
- garlic
- dill
- Romaine lettuce

Put all ingredients in a bowl and mix with your hands. Wrap in lettuce leaves and eat up

56

Dill Salad

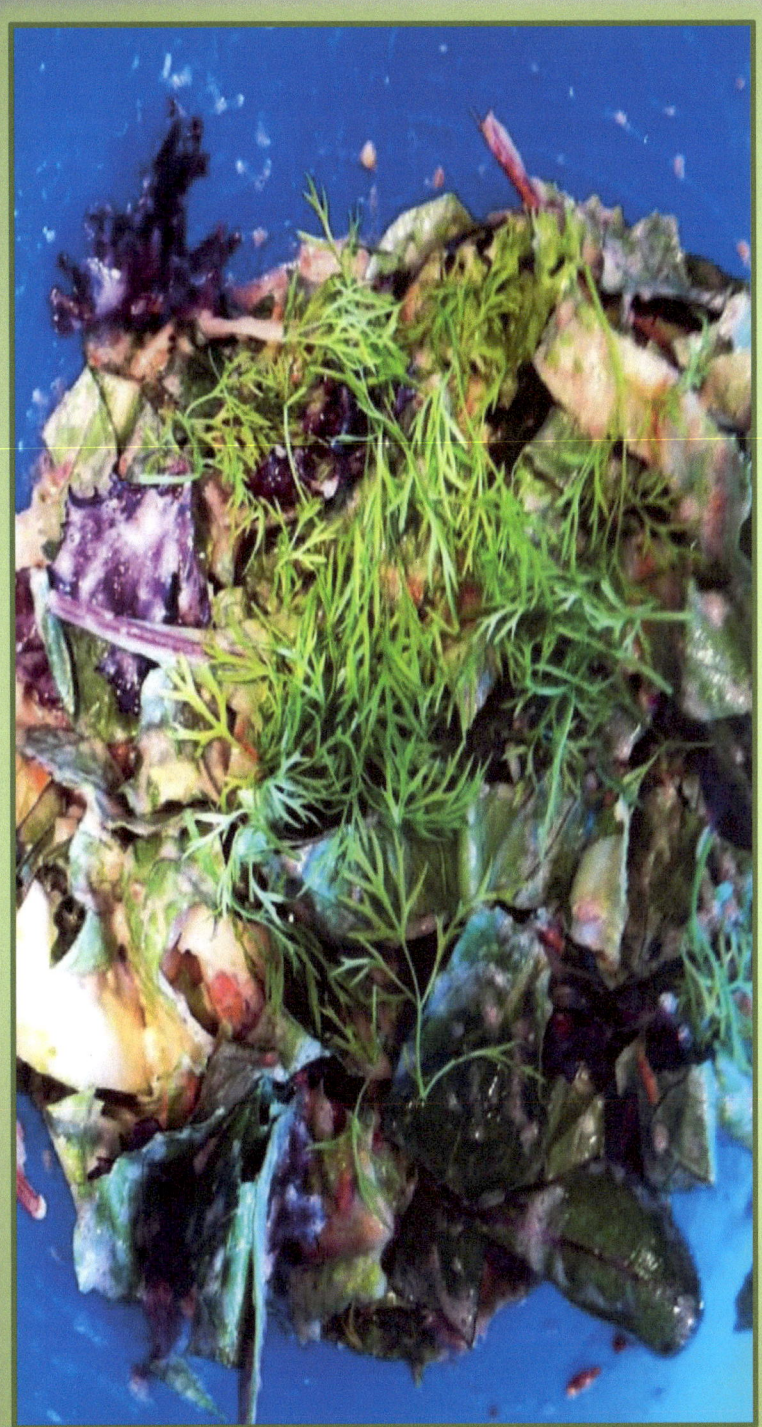

- dill
- mixed greens
- lettuce of your choice
- Tahini
- garlic
- fresh tomatoes

For the sauce

Mix tomatoes with Tahini and garlic

Mixed Salad with Mango sauce

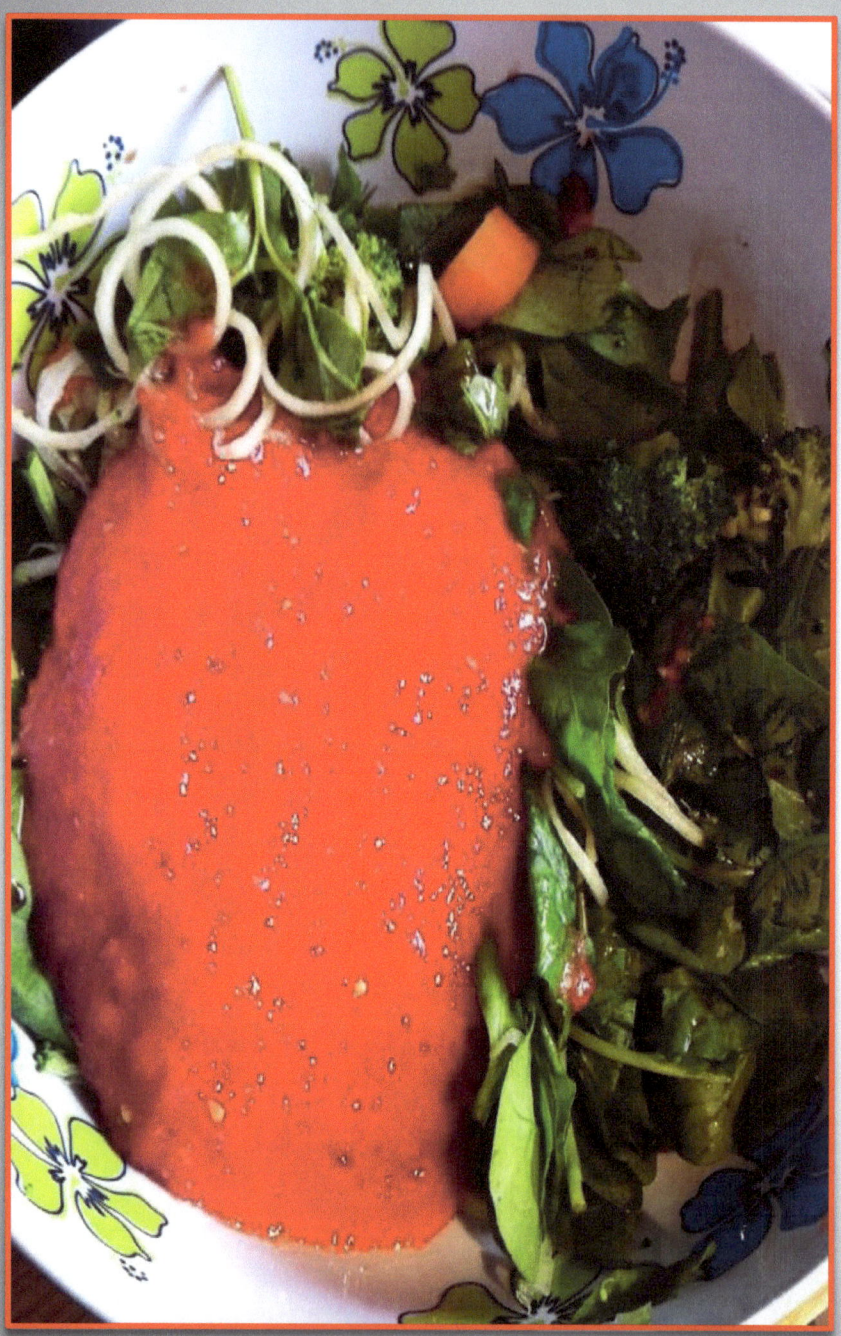

- courgette (zucchini) noodles (optional)
- mixed greens of your choice
- lettuce of your choice
- broccoli
- lemon juice

For the sauce
Mix ripe mango with red peppers

Tomato & Pepper Soup

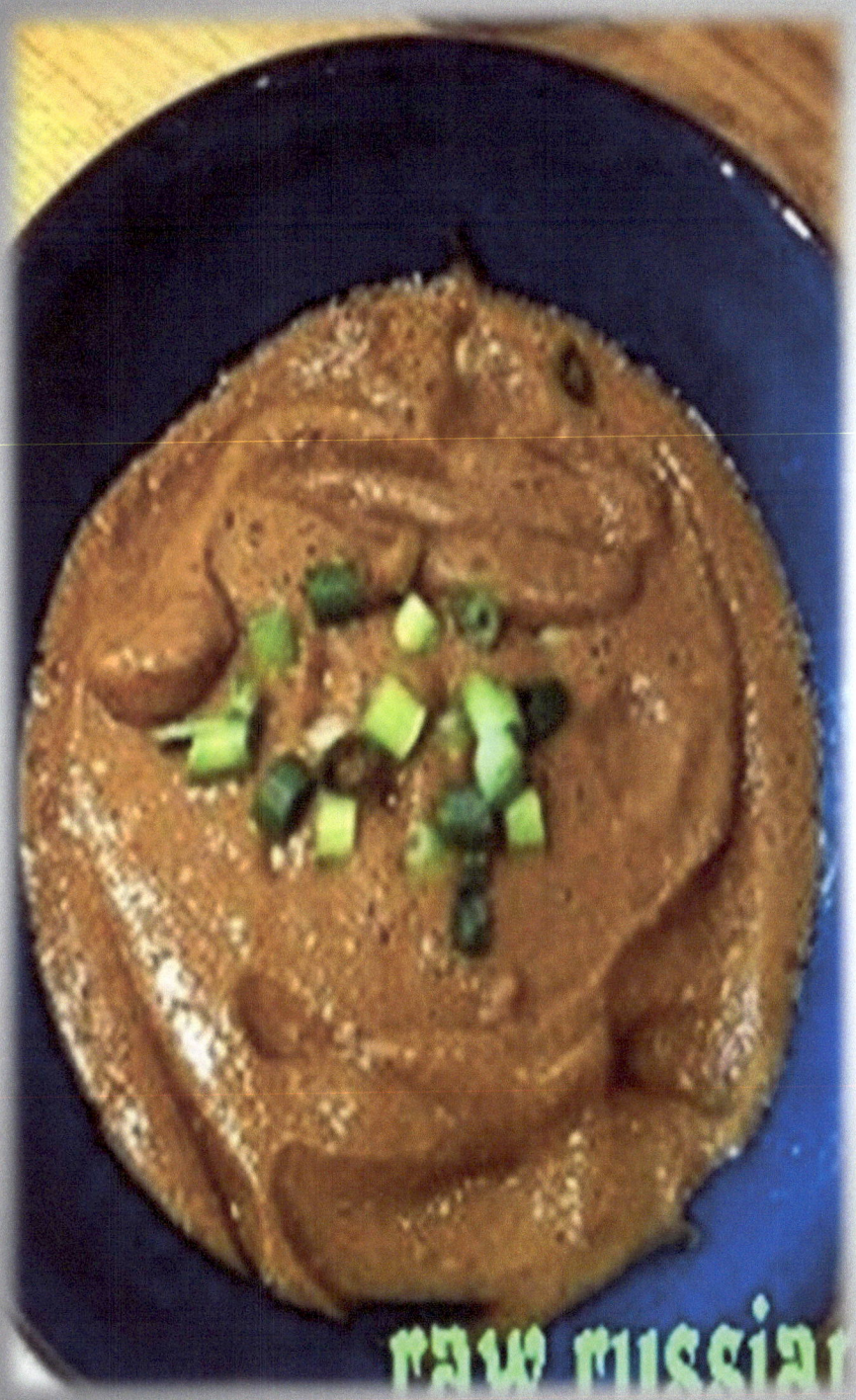

One of my absolute favourites! I can eat buckets of it

- red peppers
- tomatoes
- lemon juice
- celery
- cucumber
- avocado (optional)
- herbs of your choice

Blend it all together. Super quick and delicious

Bean Paste Snack

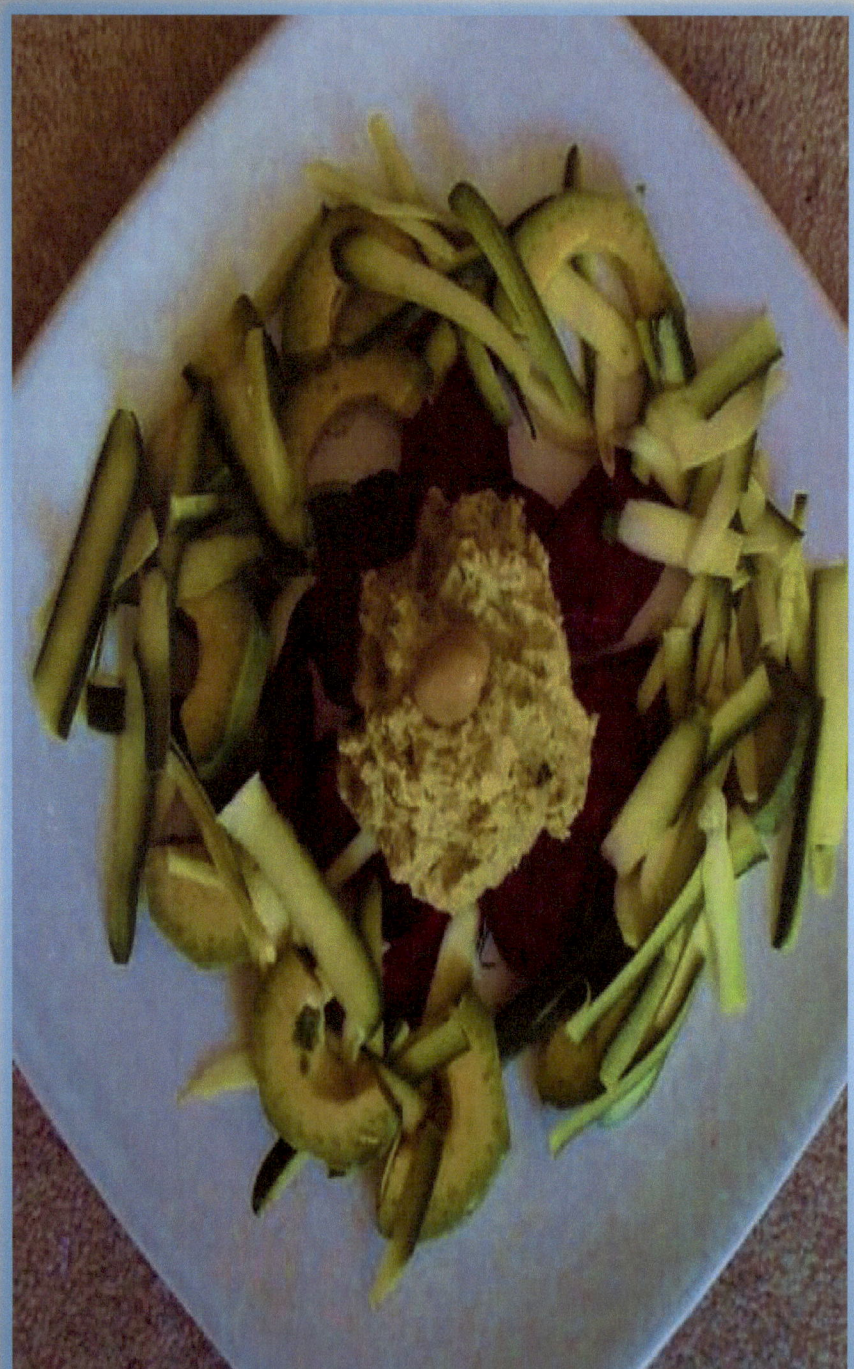

- avocado
- courgette (zucchini)
- cucumber
- beet root

Finely shred avocado, courgette, cucumber & slice beet root.

For the paste
- butter beans
- garlic
- spring onion
- lemon juice

60

Zucchini with Sauce

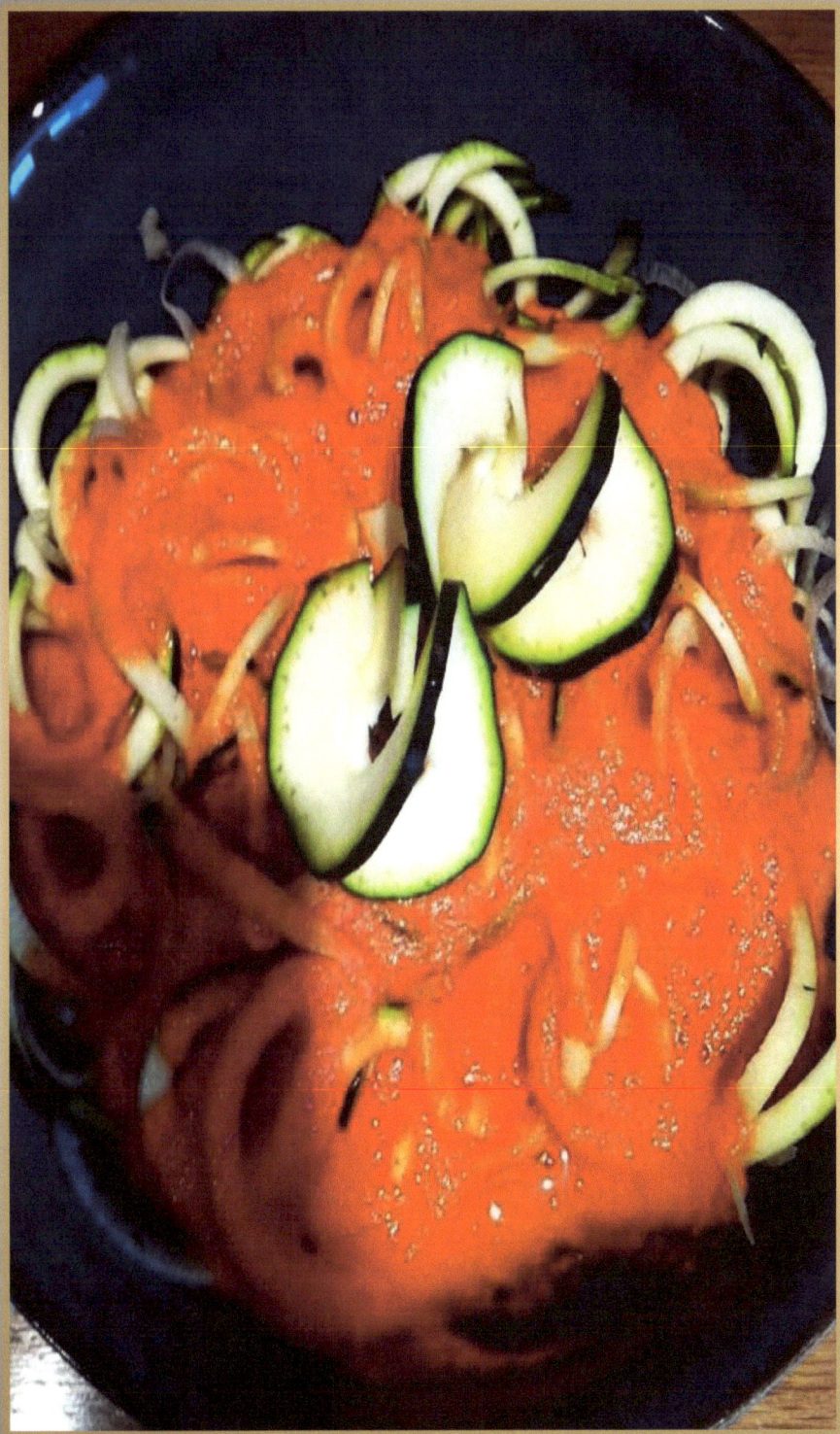

- courgette (zucchini) spiralized
- cucumber spiralized
- white onion (optional)

For the sauce
- red or yellow pepper
- celery
- tomatoes
- lemon juice

Hummus

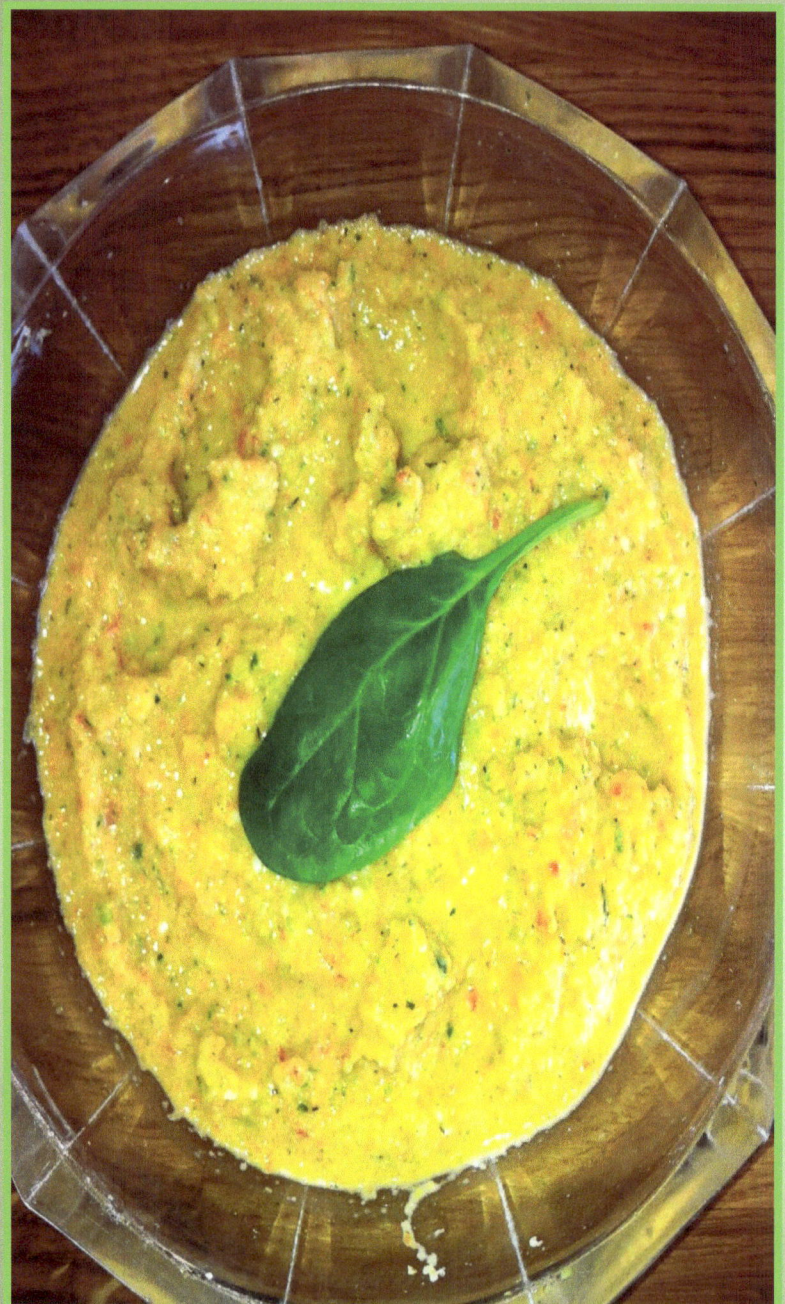

- courgette (zucchini)
- garlic
- dill
- lemon juice
- Tahini (ground sesame seeds paste)

I don't use oil in my hummus, but you are welcome to. You can also replace courgette with chickpeas or use both.

Salsa Wraps/Salad

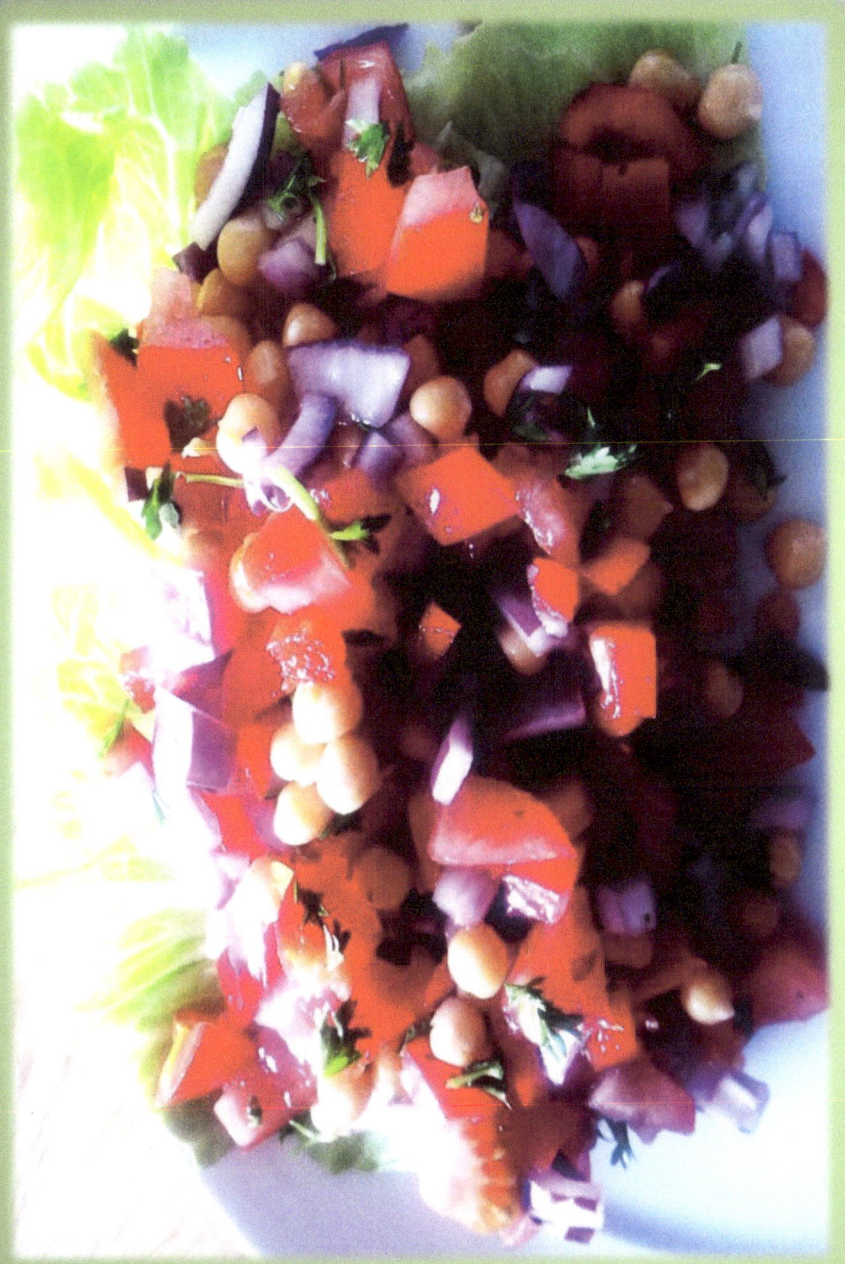

- organic chickpeas
- red onion
- fresh tomatoes
- red/green peppers
- parsley
- lime & lemon juice
- apple cider vinegar (optional)

This meal can be eaten as a salad or wrap the goodness in lettuce leaves and devour

63

Lasagne

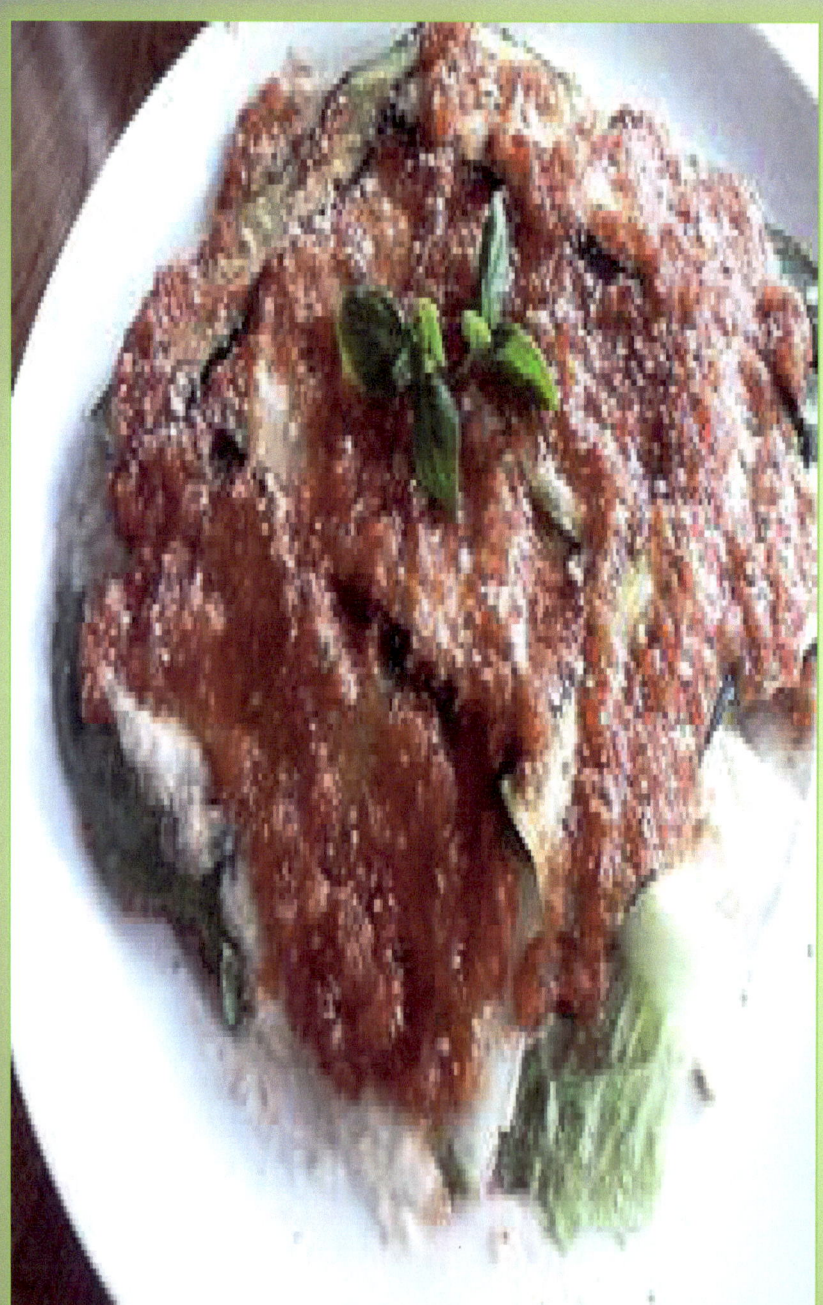

This is a low-fat version. Add pine/cashew nuts to the white sauce for a higher fat option.

Layering
- peel courgettes (using skin strips for layering)
- Romaine lettuce leaves

White sauce: (blend together)
- peeled zucchini flesh
- garlic
- celery
- chia seeds for thickness (optional, I don't normally use)
- lemon juice

Red sauce (blend together)
- basil/parsley
- tomatoes
- peppers

Sprinkle with ground almonds or finely chopped cauliflower

Citrus Salad

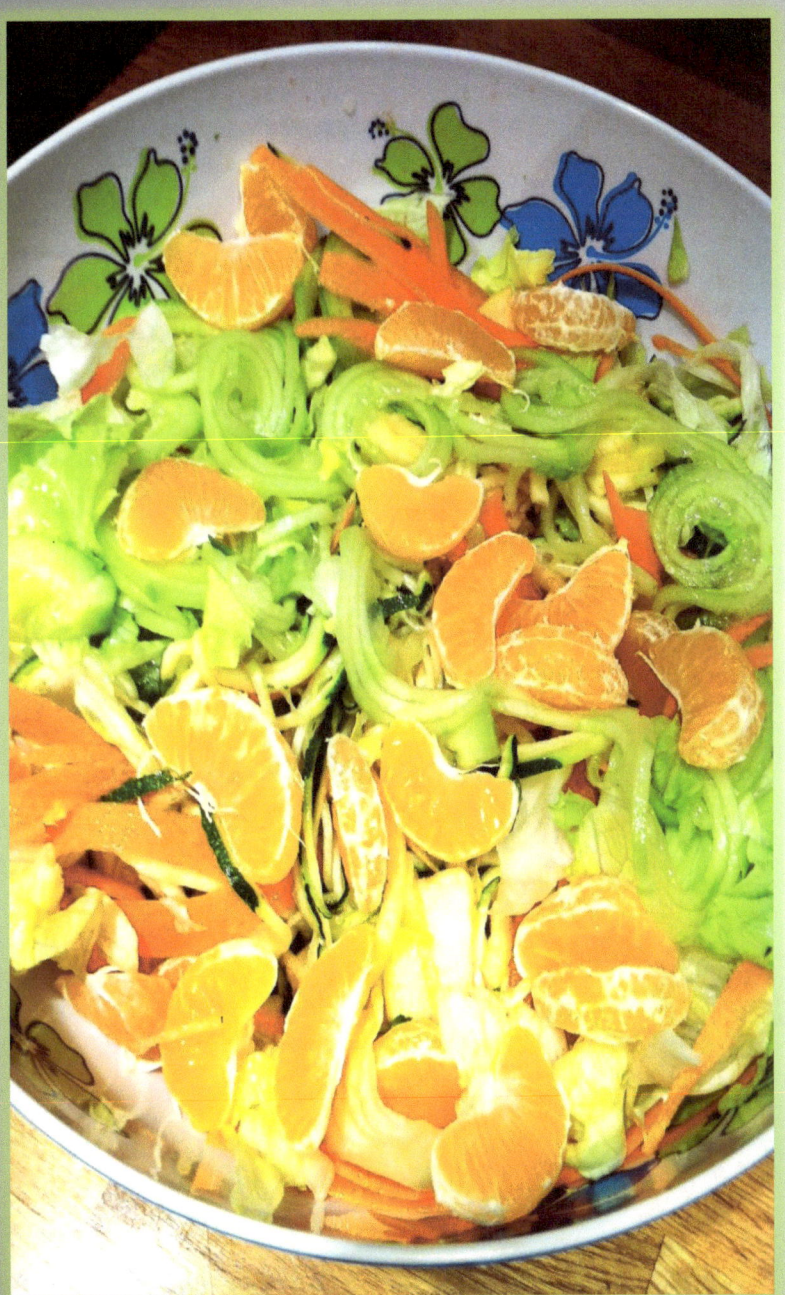

Citrus and cucumber deliciousness.
- tangerine pieces
- cucumber noodles
- courgette noodles
- shredded carrots
- romaine lettuce
- dressed in lemon juice

Very summery and fresh

Beet root Soup

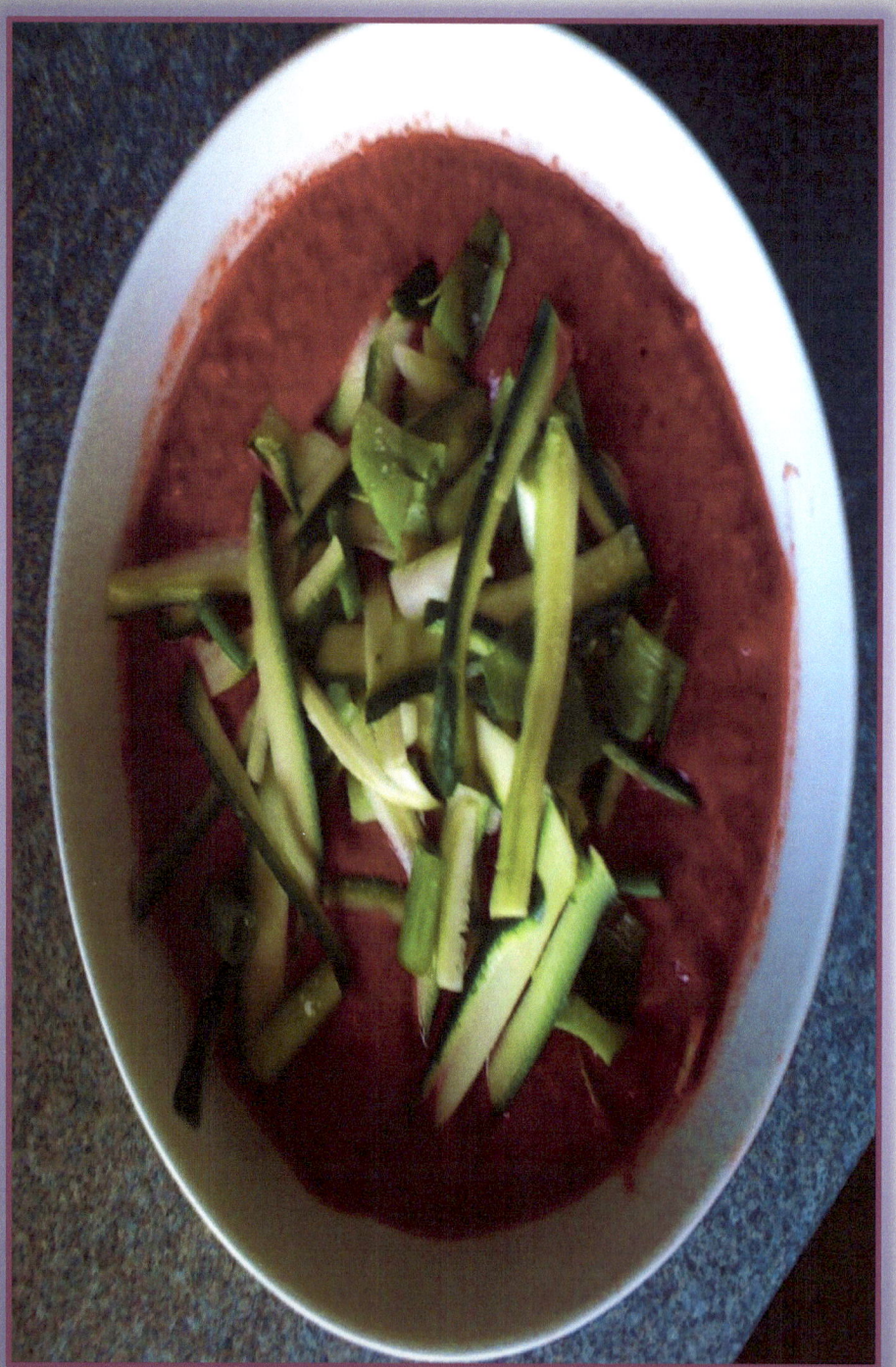

One of my favourite meals
• courgette (zucchini) shredded for garnish
• beet root
• peeled cucumber
• red pepper
• celery
• garlic
Blend all together, garnish with shredded zucchini & herbs and enjoy! Very tasty.

This soup can also be used as a dressing for a salad or over steamed vegetables

Super Greens Salad

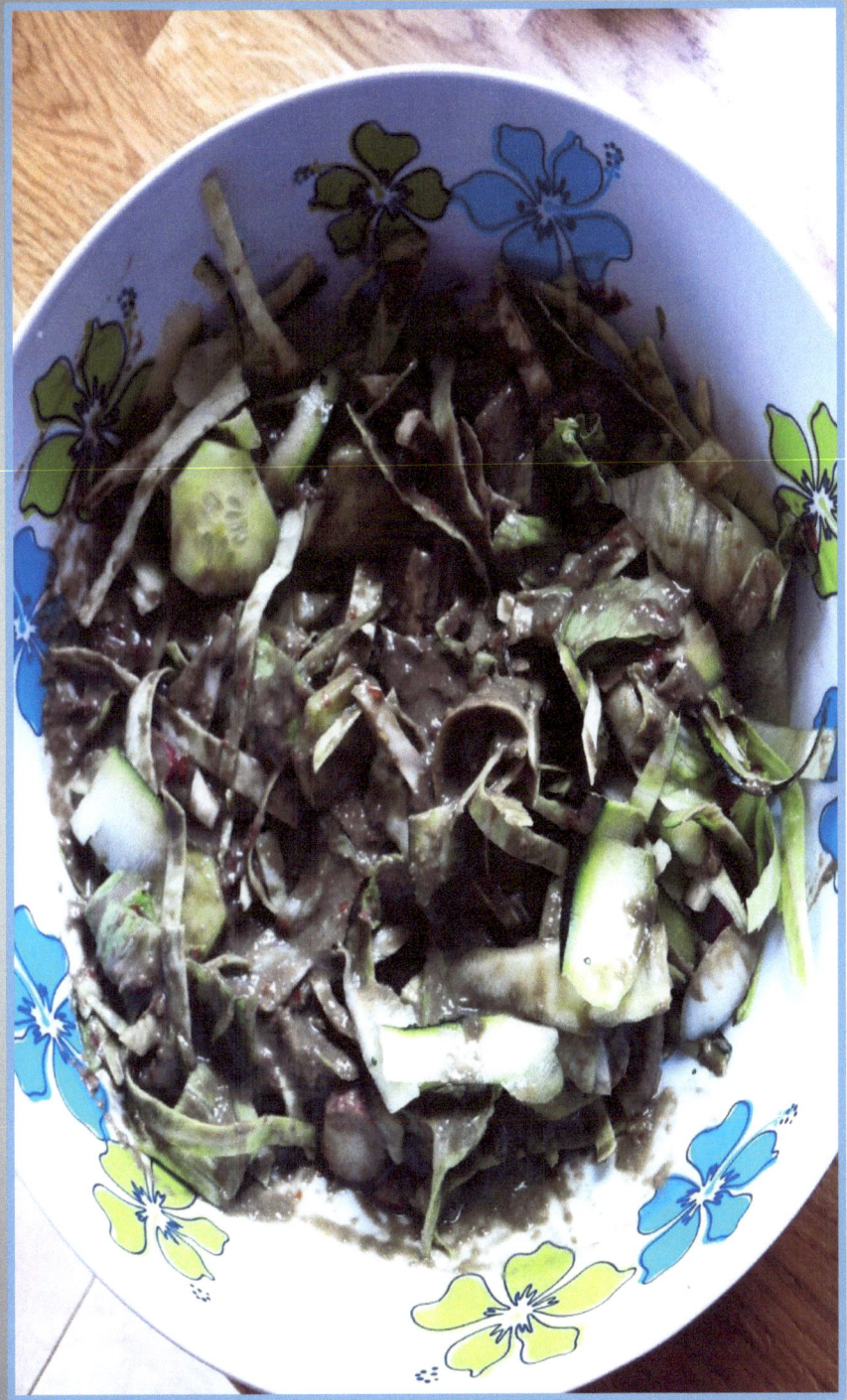

- lettuce (of your choice) or white cabbage or both
- sliced cucumbers

For the dressing
Mix together avocado, garlic, spirulina or chlorella powder. Very simple & grounding meal!

Raw Cheese

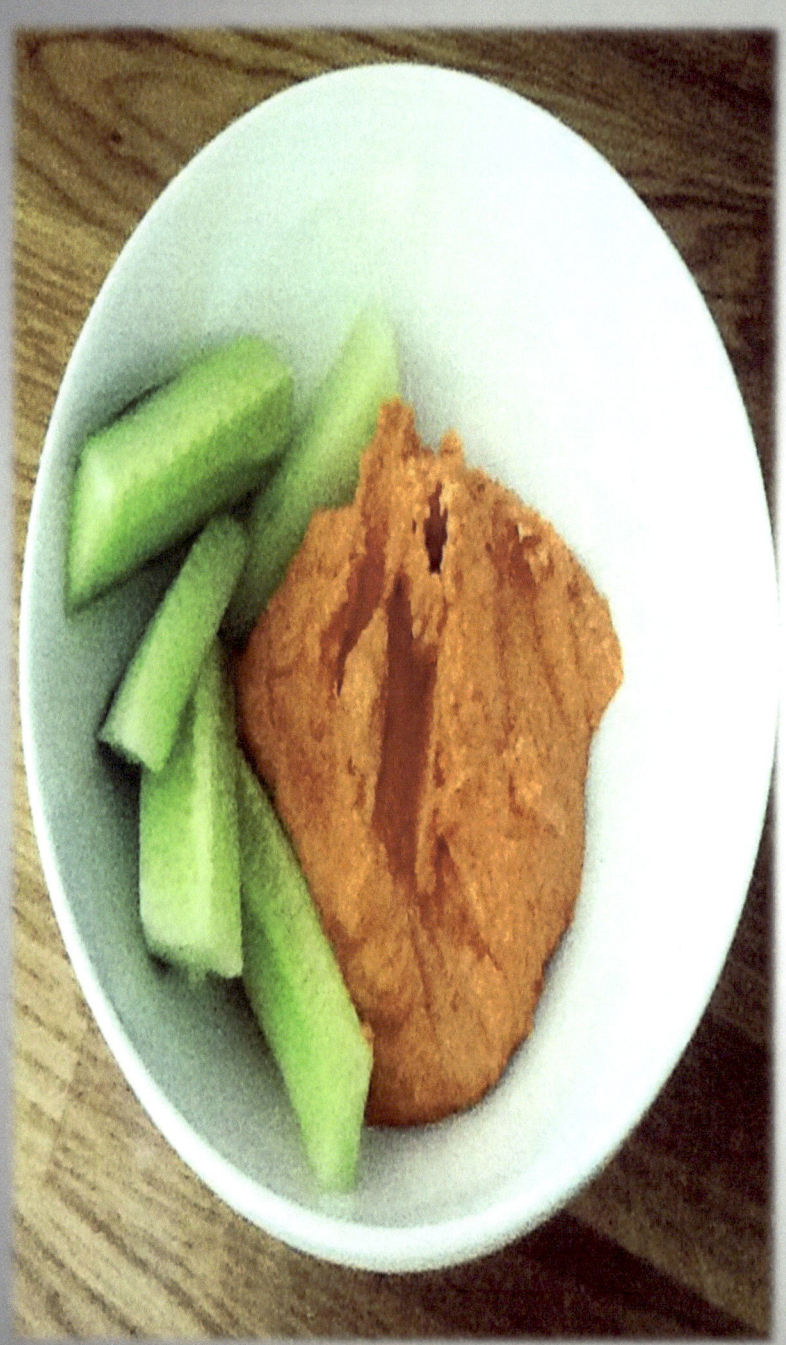

This is a high fat snack/dip

- cashew or macadamia nuts
- garlic
- red/yellow peppers

Blend all together and enjoy as a snack/dip with cucumber/carrot/pepper sticks

Beet root Boats

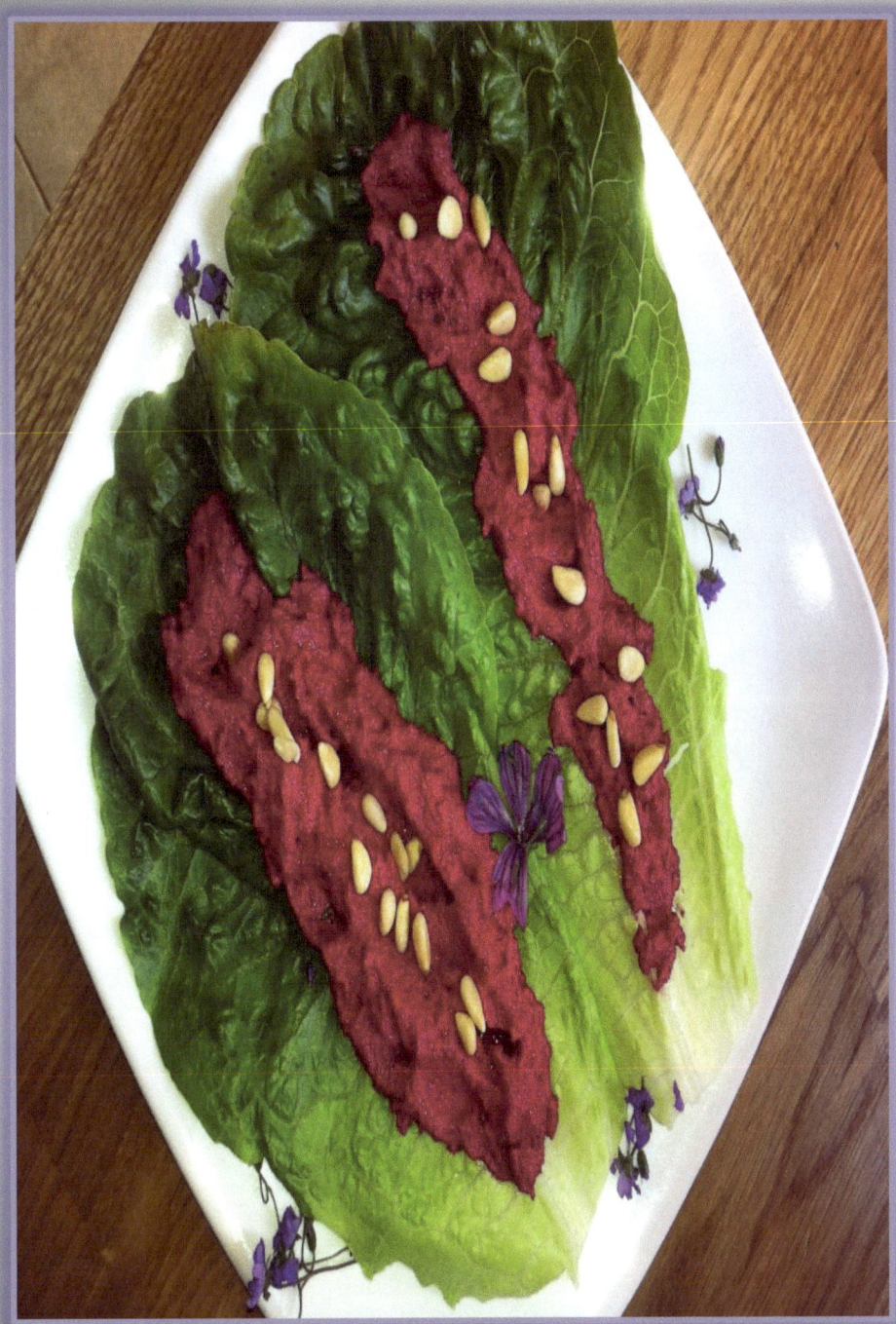

This can be eaten as a snack or a meal depending on how much you make. It is a high fat recipe. Can eat with a spoon as it is or in a lettuce wrap. Very rich in flavour

- beet root
- walnuts
- avocado
- garlic
- lemon

Blend all ingredients together, garnish with pine nuts (optional) & serve

Sprouts Salad

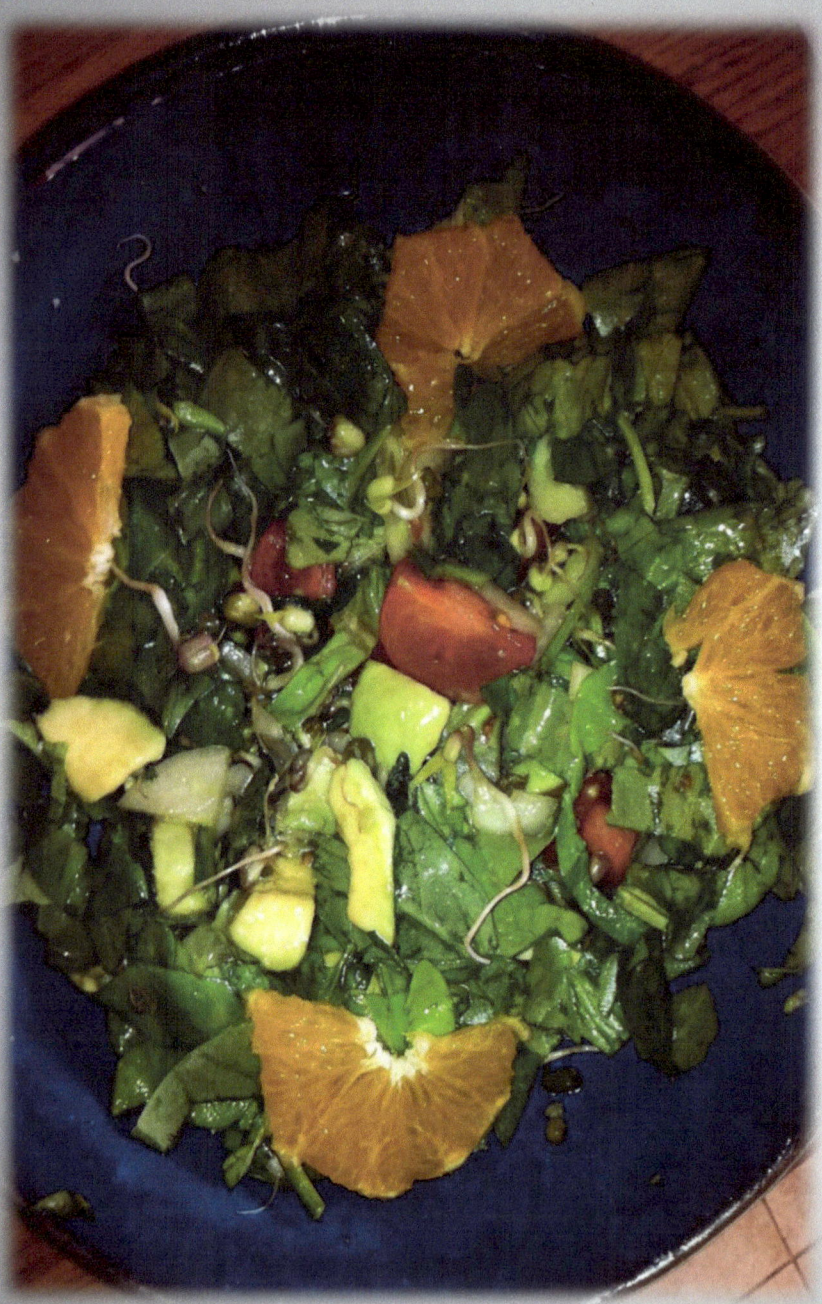

- mung bean/sunflower sprouts (can do it yourself at home)
- any greens you like
- white/red onion
- avocado
- tomatoes
- lemon & orange juice for the dressing

Zucchini Pasta

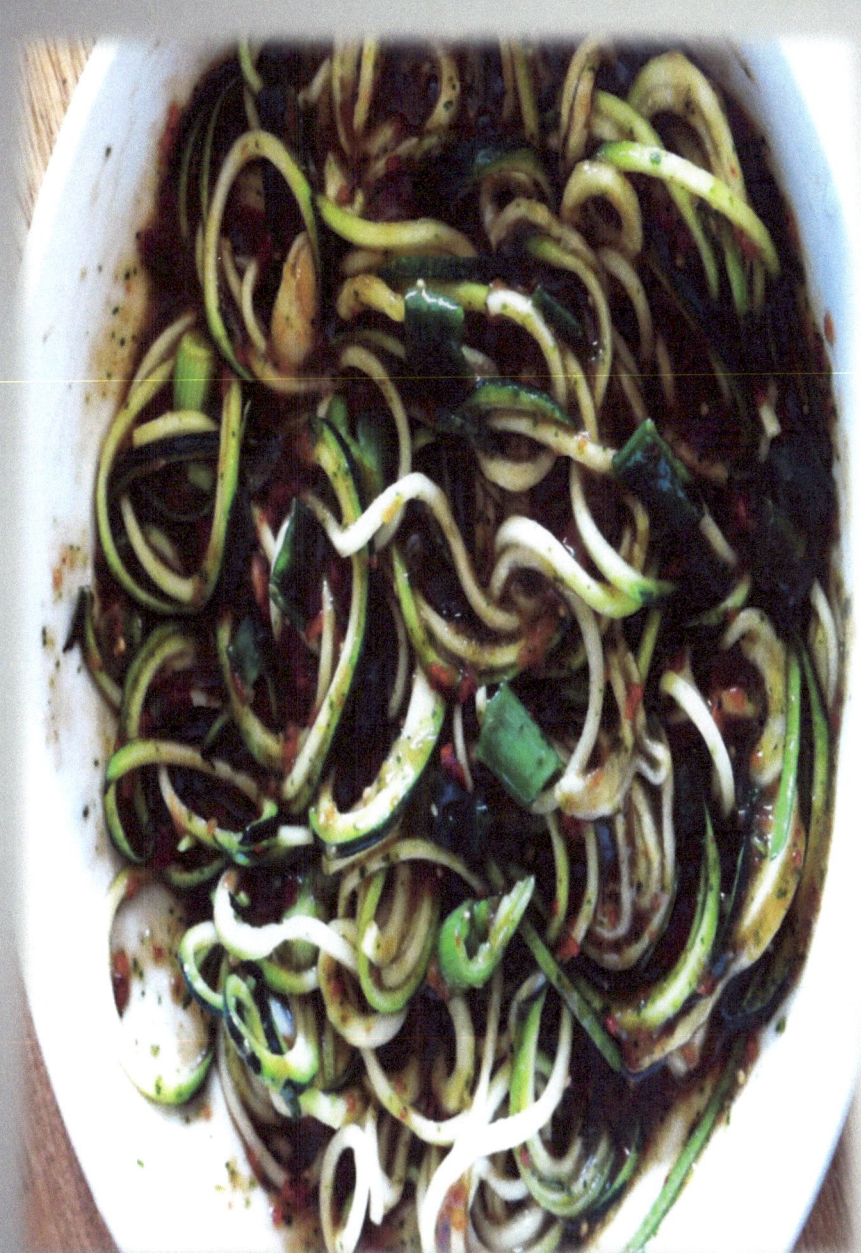

This is a meal I have very often. There are a lot of variations on the marinara sauce.

- courgette (zucchini)
- garlic (optional)
- fresh tomatoes
- celery
- red pepper
- dill
- spring onions

Spiralize some zucchini.

For the sauce:

Blend ingredients together. Mix into pasta, garnish with spring onion and enjoy. Alternatively you can simply turn this sauce into a soup and eat it as it is. You might even try adding dates or sun dried tomatoes for texture or mango and avocado for extra creaminess.

Conclusion

I hope you enjoyed my colourful display of yummy meals and feel encouraged to try them for yourself. Remember to experiment and let your creativity flow. Please visit my website for more inspiration, advice and further information about the raw lifestyle. I plan to update this book regularly, so please stay tuned for more colourful and delicious creations.

www.rawrussian.com

info@rawrussian.com